Obesity

Published by
Lotus Press

Obesity

Dr. Ramdass
Anuradha Shivkumar

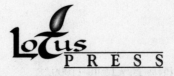

PRESS

4263/3, Ansari Road,
Darya Ganj, New Delhi-110002

LOTUS PRESS
4263/3, Ansari Road, Darya Ganj, New Delhi-110002
Ph: 30903912, 23290047, E-mail: lotus_press@sify.com

OBESITY
© 2006, Lotus Press
ISBN 81-8382-030-1

Published by: Lotus Press, New Delhi-110002
Lasertypeset by: Reliable Infomedia, New Delhi-110009
Printed at: Ashim Print Line, Delhi.

Preface

This book on obesity has been written in a very different way—not those typical "Textbook type"—which preaches high and mighty things. This book has been written not in the usual format of "cause-effect-treatment". When we are in the house we get to eat only what is in the kitchen but when we go to a cafeteria, we can get whatever we want, and of there is also the advantage of self-service. This book has been written in a cafeteria approach. Whatever one wants one can have it. Though the initial chapters briefly delineate the definitions, causes, ways to tackle obesity, once the discussion shifts to diet, exercise, research findings and special cases (pregnancy or childhood overweight) the approach is reader friendly or interactive. Illustration of pictures; snippets from fairy tales, mythology; album on obesity, have all been added to generate interest, curiosity, of awareness among readers. Students, children, common man, doctors or housewives—everybody will have something of his interest in this book.

Happy Reading   **Author**

Contents

1

Introduction

Certain Basic Principles

Obesity means deposit of excess fat in the body. It is caused by ingestion of greater amounts of food that can be utilised by the body for energy. The excess food, whether fats, carbohydrates or proteins, is then stored as fat in the adipose tissue to be used later for energy. It will be interesting to know that strains of rats have been found in which hereditary obesity occurs. In at least one of these strains the obesity is caused by ineffective mobilisation of fat from the adipose tissue while synthesis and storage of fat continue normally. Obviously such a one-way process causes progressive enhancement of the fat stores, resulting in severe obesity!

When greater quantities of energy (in the form of food) enter the body than are expended, the body weight increases. Therefore, obesity is obviously caused by an excess energy input over energy output. For each 9.3 calories of excess energy entering the body 1 gram of fat is stored.

Excess energy input occurs only during the developing phase of obesity, and once a person has become obese all that is required to remain obese is that the energy input equals the energy output. For the person to reduce weight, the input must be less than the output. Indeed studies of obese persons have shown that the intake of food in most of them in the *static stage* of obesity (after the obesity has already been attained) is approximately the same as that for normal persons.

About one-third of the energy used each day by the normal person goes into muscular activity and in the labourer as much as two-thirds or occasionally three-fourths is used in this way. Since muscular activity is by far the most important means by which energy is expended in the body, it is frequently said that obesity results from too high a ratio of food intake to daily exercise.

It is a known fact that the rate of feeding is normally regulated in proportion to the nutrients store in the body. When these stores begin to reach an optimal level in a normal person, feeding is *automatically* reduced to prevent overstorage. However, in many obese persons this is not true, for feeding does not slacken until body weight is far above normal. Therefore, in effect, obesity is often caused by an abnormality of the feeding regulatory mechanism. This can result from many factors which will be discussed in subsequent chapters.

Having defined obesity in so many words it is important to know what is the exact opposite of obesity. 'Inanition' is the opposite of obesity. In addition to inanition caused by inadequate availability of food, various psychogenic and hormonal causes can on occasion cause greatly decreased feeding. One such condition *'Anorexia Nervosa'* is an abnormal psychic state in which a person loses all desire for food and even becomes nauseated by it; as a result *inanition* occurs. Certain destructive lesions of the hypothalamus (regulation centre of brain) cause a condition called *Cachexia*. The term simply means severe inanition.

Cause for Concern

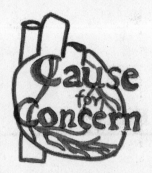

Obesity is defined as being 20% or more over ideal body weight. It increases the risk of heart disease and diabetes. It is known to cause serious health problems. Increasing body weight is associated with increasing blood cholesterol levels, high BP and decreased levels of HDL (good cholesterol) and physical inactivity. According to the National Centre for Health Statistics BMI is recommended to be not more than 25. If BMI exceeds 25 there is an increased risk of developing heart disease and other illnesses associated with being overweight!

Did she have Anorexia or Bulemia Nervosa?

The late Princess Diana was often said to be suffering from Anorexia Nervosa. In fact, her complete lack of desire for food was attributed to *Bulemia,* a condition characterised by eating and later vomitting—a kind of psychic state.

The cycles of eating and purging are self-induced. Diana also had water treatment or hydrotherapy every week when she took litres and litres of water (as enema) to clear and cleanse her system!

How much of all these were true and how much were rumours, only God knows!

Recent studies link anorexia nervosa and polycystic ovarian disease. A lot of new and important information on this topic is being published in medical journals.

2

Hard-hitting Facts

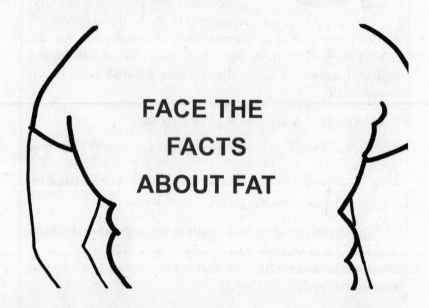

FACE THE
FACTS
ABOUT FAT

Face the Facts About Fat

1. You don't have to look fat to suffer from its effects. Being even slightly overweight can put you at increased risk of many serious health problems.

2. Fat is the culprit. Combined with a lack of exercise, a high fat diet is the basic cause of obesity and weight gain. Obesity, or being overweight, is associated with health

4

problems such as stroke, heart disease, arthritis, certain types of cancer and premature death. Being overweight also puts you at risk of conditions such as high blood pressure and type 2 diabetes.

What is the easiest way to lose weight? There is no easy way to lose weight. Health care professionals agree that weight loss is best achieved by following a healthy diet and taking regular exercises. However, if these measures are unsuccessful, your doctor may consider the use of medication for weight loss. There are two kinds of medication currently available— those which suppress appetite and those which inhibit fat absorption.

Your doctor can help you. He talk to your doctor before going on a weight loss programme so that can advise you on appropriate methods to lose weight and maintain a healthy weight.

The slogan to remember is: "Lose Weight, Gain Life."

Big is beautiful. This applies to a majestic elephant; a big heart which means a generous, magnanimous, benevolent, forgiving, noble heart; a broad mind having tolerant views, but a 'big mouth' or a big body (obesity) is definitely not beautiful or healthy. Remember when you control your body weight you become both healthy and beautiful.

Whatever be the weight-reducing method—appetite suppressants, fat burners, weight-reducing machines, gels— the method must be:

1. workable on a long-term basis

2. to not strain your will power

3. to not risk your health.

When an obese woman begins to work hard and loses weight it is not that she will immediately become pencil thin or she will get an hour-glass figure. She may still be on the

large side but control of the weight is the most important factor.
When she achieves this she feels great.

Obesity Perils

World over 17 crore 60 lakh people suffer from diabetes;
of this:

- 80 per cent are due to obesity!
- 40 per cent uterine and cervical cancers.
- 25 per cent kidney, urinary, bladder etc. cancers.
- 10 per cent breast cancers are due to obesity.
- 21 percent heart diseases (coronary heart diseases).

Not all that is Big is Beautiful

Big and Beautiful

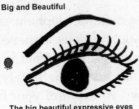

The big, beautiful, expressive eyes

Big...,
but definitely not
beautiful!

A fat
obese
body

**Big heart
(Generous,
magnanimous
heart)**

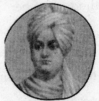

**The Big -
'broad mind'**

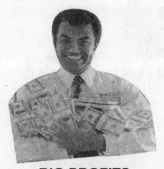

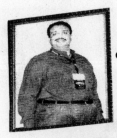

An
overweight,
unhealthy
physique

BIG PROFITS
BIG MONEY
BIG DISCOUNTS
BIG DEALS
BIG BUILDINGS &
MONUMENTS
Big chance
Big show

Big Blow

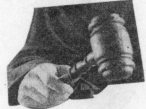

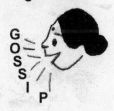

The huge
majestic
elephant
'all big, all powerful'

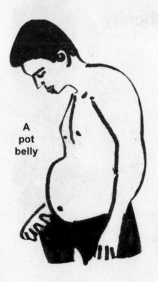

A big mouth

G
O
S
S
I
P

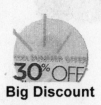

A
pot
belly

30% OFF
Big Discount

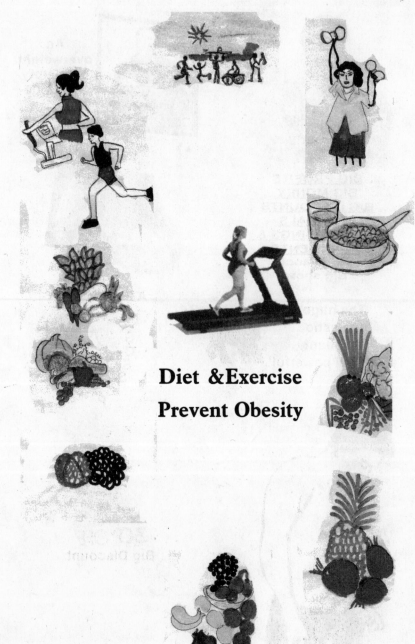

Diet &Exercise
Prevent Obesity

3

Dietary Balances

The intake of food must always be sufficient to supply the metabolic needs of the body and yet not so much as to cause obesity. Since different foods contain different proportions of proteins, carbohydrates, fats, an appropriate balance must be maintained among these different types of food so that all segments can be supplied with the requisite materials.

The energy liberated from each gram of carbohydrate as it is oxidised to carbon dioxide and water is 4.1 calories (cal), and that liberated from fat is 9.3 calories. The energy liberated from metabolism of the average protein of the diet as each gram is oxidised to carbon dioxide, water and urea is 4.35 calories. Also these different substances vary in the average percentages that are absorbed from the gastrointestinal : tract approximately 98% of carbohydrate, 95% of the fat, 92% of the protein. Therefore, the average physiologically available energy in each gram of the three different foodstuffs in the diet is:

Calories (in round figures)

Carbohydrates	4.0
Fat	9.0
Proteins	4.0

9

Average Americans receives approximately 15% of their energy from protein, 40% from fat and 45% from carbohydrates. In most of the other parts of the world the quantity of energy derived from carbohydrates far exceeds that derived from both proteins and fats. Indeed, in Mongolia, the energy received from the fat and proteins combined is said to be not greater than 15 to 20%.

High proportions of fats and proteins are present in meat products and high proportions of carbohydrates are seen in vegetables and grain products. Fat is deceptive in the diet for it usually exists as 100% fat whereas both proteins and carbohydrates are mixed in watery media so that each of these normally represents less than 25% of the weight as food. Therefore, the fat of one pat of butter mixed with an entire helping of potatoes often contains as much energy as all the potato itself.

Daily Requirement of Protein

Twenty to 30 gms of the body proteins are degraded and used for producing other body chemicals daily. Therefore, all cells must continue to form new proteins to take the place of those that are being destroyed, and a supply of protein is needed in the diet for this purpose. An average person can maintain normal stores of protein provided the daily intake is above 30 to 55 gms. In general, proteins derived from animal foodstuffs are more nearly complete than are proteins derived from the vegetable and grain sources. Animal proteins have all the amino acids whereas many of the vegetable or grain proteins are only partial proteins.

Carbohydrates and Fats as 'Protein Sparesr'

When the diet contains an abundance of carbohydrates and fats almost all the body's energy is derived from these two substances and very little is derived from the proteins. Therefore, both carbohydrates and fats are said to be protein sparers. On the other hand, in starvation after the carbohydrate and fats have been depleted the body's protein stores are then consumed rapidly for energy, sometimes at rates approaching several hundred grams per day rather than at the normal daily rate of 30 to 55 gms.

Regulation of Food Intake

1. **Hunger:** The term 'Hunger' means a craving for food and it is associated with a number of objective sensations. For instance, in a person who has not had food for many hours the stomach undergoes intense rhythmic contractions called *hunger contractions*. These cause a tight or gnawing feeling in the pit of the stomach and sometimes actually cause pain called *hunger pangs*. In addition to the hunger pangs the hungry person also becomes more tense and restless than usual.

    Some physiologists actually define hunger as contractions of the stomach. However, even after the hunger is completely removed the psychic sensations of hunger still occur and craving for food still makes the person search for an adequate food supply.

2. **Appetite:** The term 'appetite' is often used in the same sense as hunger except that it usually implies a desire for specific types of food instead of food in general. Therefore, an appetite helps a person choose the quality of food to eat.

3. **Satiety:** Satiety is the opposite of hunger. It means a feeling of fulfilment in the quest for food. Satiety usually results from a full meal, particularly when the person's nutritional storage depots, the adipose tissue and the glycogen stores are already filled.

Neural Centres for Regulation of Food Intake

Hunger and satiety centres are located in the hypothalamus, one of the very important centres of brain. The lateral nuclei of the hypothalamus is named as the *hunger* centre or feeding centre, and ventromedial nuclei of the hypothalamus is termed as *satiety centre*. The feeding centre operates by directly exciting the emotional drive to search for food. On the other hand, it is believed that the satiety centre operates primarily by inhibiting the feeding centre. Certain important areas of brain like limbic system also control feeding appetite.

The important factors that regulate food intake are:

1. *Nutritional regulation* : This is primarily concerned with the maintenance of normal quantities of nutrient stores in the body. Availability of glucose to the body cells, amino acid concentration in blood, fat metabolites (adipose tissue quantity) all regulate feeding. This regulation is called long-term regulation.

2. *Alimentary regulation* : This is concerned primarily with the immediate effects of feeding on the alimentary tract and is sometimes called peripheral regulation or short-term regulation. Gastro intestinal filling, factors relating to chewing, salivation, swallowing and fasting are the various alimentary regulation principles regulating food intake.

Starvation

Except for the first few hours of starvation (when carbohydrate is depleted) the major effects are progressive depletion of tissue fat and protein. Since fat is the prime source of energy its rate of depletion continues unabated, until most of the fat stores in the body are gone. Protein undergoes three different phases of deletion:

1. Rapid depletion at first.

2. Then greatly slowed depletion.

3. Finally rapid depletion again shortly before death.

Vitamin deficiencies in starvation : The stores of some of the vitamins, especially the water soluble vitamins B and C, do not last long during starvation. After a week of starvation mild vitamin deficiencies usually begin to appear, and after several weeks severe vitamin deficiencies can occur. These can add to the debility that leads to death.

For crazy youngsters who go to the extreme levels—like starvation—to become trim and slim, the above facts will be a real eye opener.

4

Abnormal Feeding Regulation

The rate of feeding is normally regulated in proportion to the nutrient stores in the body. When these stores begin to approach an optimal level in a normal person, feeding is automatically reduced to prevent overstorage. However, in many obese persons this is not true, for feeding does not slacken until body weight is far above normal. Therefore, in effect, obesity is often caused by an abnormality of the feeding regulatory mechanism. This can result from either the psychogenic factors that affect the regulation or actual abnormalities of the hypothalamus self.

1.Psychogenic Obesity

Studies of obese patients show that a large proportion of obesity results from psychogenic factors. The most common psychogenic factor contributing to obesity is the prevalent idea that healthy eating habits require three meals a day and that each meal must be filling. Many children are forced into this habit by overly solicitous parents and the children continue to practise it throughout life. In addition, persons are known often to gain large amounts of weight during or following stressful situations such as death of a parent, a severe illness, or even mental depression. It seems that eating is often a means of release from tension.

2.Hypothalamic Abnormalities

Hypothalamus, the higher centres of the brain, is concerned with regulation of food intake. Lesions in the ventromedial nuclei of the hypothalamus cause an animal to eat excessively and become obese. It has also been discovered that such lesions are associated with excess insulin production which in-turn increases fat deposition. Also many persons with hypophysical tumours that encroach on the hypothalamus develop progressive obesity, illustrating that obesity in the human being, too, can definitely result from damage to the hypothalamus.

Yet in the normal obese person hypothalamic damage is almost never found. Nevertheless it is possible that the functional organisation of the feeding centre is different in the obese person from that of the non-obese person. For instance, a normally obese person who has reduced to normal weight by strict dietary measures usually develops hunger that is demonstrably for greater than that of the normal person. This indicates that the 'set point' of the obese persons feeding centre is at a much higher level of nutrient storage than that of the normal person.

3.Genetic Factors

Obesity definitely runs in families. Furthermore, identical twins usually maintain weight levels within two pounds of each other throughout life if they live under similar conditions or within five pounds of each other if their conditions of life differ markedly. This might result partly from eating habits engendered during childhood, but it is generally believed that this close similarity between twins is genetically controlled.

The genes can direct the degree of feeding in several different ways including a genetic abnormality of the feeding centre to set the level of nutrient storage high or low, abnormal hereditary psychic factors that either whet the appetite or cause the person to eat as a 'release' mechanisn.

'LEPTIN'—Its role in body fat control and puberty

Leptin—This chemical was identified several years ago as a protein secreted by adipose cells that tells the adult body "STOP eating, you are fat enough". Levels of leptin in blood also initiates puberty, says the new research findings. Leptin seems to be the main signal that reflects to the brain the amount of fat, the individual has accumulated. Human studies reveal that only because of these leptin signals, chubby girl of 10 go through the puberty early and thin athletic girls are delayed in their onset of mensuration. Leptin helps orchestrate puberty in males also.

Experiments in mice reveal that genetically allotted mice become obese when the leptin lacks in their body (due to genetic alterations).

This is because they are deprived of leptin signals to stop eating. In addition, they also become sterile; when leptin was supplied their fertility was restored. Leptin, thus by controlling body fat, seems to regulate puberty. Experiments are being conducted in mice and the researchers are trying to explain the findings by applying them to human beings.

In female mice, if leptin injections were given experimentally, it signalled premature puberty and even reproduction!

Thus the role of leptin in "Fat Control" in body and puberty is becoming more and more prominent.

Genetic abnormalities in the chemistry of fat storage are also known to cause absentee in certain strains of rats and mice. In one strain of rats, fat is easily stored in the adipose tissue but the quantity of hormone sensitive lipase in the adipose tissue is greatly reduced, so that little of fat can be removed. In addition, these rats develop hyperinsulinism (insulin) which also promotes fat storage. This combination obviously results in a one-way path, the fat continually being deposited but never released. In a strain of obese mice that has been studied, there is excess of 'fatty acid syntheses', which causes excess synthesis of fatty acids. Thus, similar genetic mechanisms are other possible causes of obesity in human beings.

4.Childhood Overnutrition

The rate of formation of new fat cells is especially rapid in the first few years of life, and the greater the rate of fat storage the greater also becomes the number of fat cells. In obese children the number of fat cells is often as much as three times that in normal children. However, after adolescence the number of fat cells remain almost identically the same throughout the remainder of life. Therefore, it has been suggested that overfeeding the children, especially in infancy and to a lesser extent during the older years of childhood, can lead to a lifetime of obesity. The person who has excess fat cells is thought to have a higher setting of fat storage by the hypothalamic feedback auto regulatory mechanism for adipose tissues. In less obese persons, especially those who become obese in middle or old age, most of the obesity results from hyperbiophy (enlargement) of already existing fat cells. This type of obesity is far more susceptible to treatment than is the life long type. An interesting peculiarity of this type of obesity is that these persons have excess secretion of insulin, similar to the excess insulin secretion that occurs in animals with lesions in the ventromedial nuclei of the hypothalamus.

Treatment of Obesity

Treatment depends simply on decreasing energy input below energy expenditure. In other words, this means partial starvation. For this purpose most diets are designed to contain large quantities of 'bulk' which in general are made up of non-nutritive cellulose substances. This bulk distends the stomach and thereby partially appeases the hunger. In most lower animals such a procedure simply makes the animal increase its food intake still further, but human beings can often fool themselves because their food intake is sometimes controlled as much by habit as by hunger. As pointed out by all the diet experts the important point to remember is to prevent vitamin deficiencies during the dieting period. Various drugs for decreasing the degree of hunger have been used in the treatment of obesity. The most important of these is amphetamine (or amphetamine derivatives) which directly inhibits the feeding centre in the lateral nuclei of hypothalamus. However, there is danger in using this drug because it simultaneously over-excites the central nervous system making the person nervous and elevating the blood pressure. Also a person soon adapts to the drug so that weight reduction is usually no greater than 10 per cent. Finally, the more exercise one takes, the greater is the daily energy expenditure and the more rapidly the obesity disappears. Therefore, forced exercise is often an essential part of the treatment for obesity.

5

Those Numbers on the Scale

Sometimes when a person weighs himself on the weighing scale he finds that he weighs more than what he did, before he started the health programme. Often a person thinks that the whole idea of eating less and exercising is to lose weight. When he goes to the gym there are basically only two things he cares about: gaining muscle and losing weight. That's all. Of course there is the question of his health too. But if one loses fat and gains muscle, good health usually comes with it.

Most people are not aware how much fat they are losing and how much muscle they are gaining. All that matters to them is the weight loss on the weighing scales. When a person decides to measure his physical progress he should never use the scale as an indicator. A person's weight does not reflect how healthy he is or the progress he has made. When a person steps on the scale, his weight reflects the combined total of both his lean body weight (muscle, bone, organs, fluids) and body fat weight.

People are so unconvinced that they continue to be obsessed over silly numbers on the scale again and again. For the most part they do so out of ignorance. After all, the scale has been our one and only guide. Unfortunately the scale can be extremely misleading. Body composition is what matters!

Therefore if a person is eating right and exercising appropriately he need not be alarmed if his scale shows an increase in weight. *Gaining weight need not necessarily mean one is getting fat!*

When he begins his fitness programme, he will add muscle which causes his weight to increase. This will elevate his metabolism however which causes loss of body fat as well as inches. That is why one should never be discouraged if one's weight either stays the same or increases.

If a person is not concerned with the type of weight he loses, the scales are fine but if he wants to and wishes to improve his appearance they serve no purpose alone.

From the above discussion one must be able to understand the value of weighing scales. How the readings are to be interpreted becomes clear from the explanations given above. Whenever you take up an exercise or diet programme and want some kind of weight reduction it is better that you read a bit on the subject. A knowledge of concepts as discussed above gives a clear perception and you will be able to interpret the results with clarity.

Fat Percentages in a Man and Woman

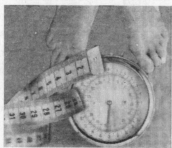

In the body of an average adult man (young age) the percentage of fat is 6 to 9%.

In the body of an average adult woman (young age) the percentage of fat is 12 to 16%.

6

The Correct Goal

What should a person's (aspiring for fitness) real goal be? Weight loss or inch loss, we see it everywhere: Lose 10 kilos, 'Turn fat into muscle', 'Trim inches from your waistline'—health club advertisements carry such slogans. Do these statements make sense? Are they possible? One can lose 10 kilos of body weight. One can make the circumference of his waist smaller, but one *cannot* turn fat into muscle. It is not physically possible. Should a person's goal be to lose kilos of body weight?

Our bodies are made up of muscle and fat. We must have a certain percentage of fat in order for us to even survive. Of course, most of us have that percentage plus quite a few percentage points more. When many people make weight loss their number one goal they often starve themselves or take to aerobics like there is no tomorrow.

What happens when one starves? We have discussed a bit about it. First our body starts to use our fat stores and muscle stores for energy because we are not bringing in enough food to support life. Next, our body's metabolism or the rate at which it burns calories begins to slow. Our body figures that it is not getting enough food to support life, so it better to start conserving what it has stored away so that it can survive.

Our body will conserve our fat and burn our muscle for the energy it needs. Muscle takes energy to preserve our body. If it can get rid of some of that muscle then it can conserve more energy. Second, our body thinks it does not need the excess muscle anyway because it is never put under a whole lot of resistance on stress.

We have eaten like a bird and done a ton of cardiovascular exercises and lost 10 kilos. But what have we done? We have lost (most likely) about 2 kilos of fat and 8 kilos of lean muscle. That is a horrible 10 kilos of weight loss. By losing muscle our metabolism is slower. Our body burns fewer calories. Then if we go back to a normal way of eating (instead of like a bird), we will get fatter faster!

So what should our real goal be? To lose body fat. To lose the inches. Fat takes up four times more space than muscle. So how can we lose the inches? A combination of weight training with cardiovascular training gives best results. One must eat at least six small meals a day.

7

Importance of Regular Exercise

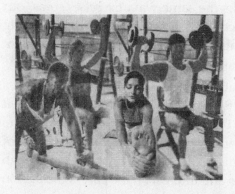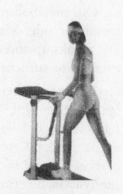

Exercise must be made a daily habit. Regular, moderate physical exercise is good for the body, mind and spirit. It reduces the possibility of coronary disease, lowers blood pressure, raises the good HDL cholesterol, helps to control weight and cuts the risk of diabetes. It helps protect against stroke, osteoporosis, and certain types of cancer. And many people regularly turn to exercise to reduce stress. These are some compelling reasons to exercise every day. Why every day? looms the question because that makes it a habit. We never remind ourselves to brush our teeth every day. It is simply a learned habit. Exercise can become one to ninety-nine per cent of the things one does each day and done on 'automatic pilot'—without consciously thinking, deciding, choosing or exerting will power. That is the power of habit, and exercise is one of the most positive habits one will ever develop.

Why else is daily exercise a good idea? Because one develops *metabolic momentum*. Our metabolism is like a spinning top. Once you twist the top it starts spinning at maximum velocity. But not long after our finger leaves contact with the top, it starts   slowing down and eventually the revolutions decrease and the top starts to wobble. One has to spin it again before it loses all its momentum and topples over. By spinning it more frequently, the average revolutions per minute stay higher and the top never slows to a wobble.

Our metabolism works the same way. Exercise 'spins' our metabolic rate. Many factors affect metabolism but nothing else cranks up and maintains our metabolic speed like frequent exercise of sufficient intensity.

To make exercise a habit it needs to be on the agenda in a specific time slot. There is no magic number for how long it takes habits to take hold. But it can happen as quickly as six to eight weeks. Once a person starts feeling the benefits of exercise, it will become his lifestyle. There should be enough motivation, determination and interest on the part of the person to make exercise a routine, daily habit. Once this happens 'fitness' comes very easily.

8

Cardio Exercises : Facts

Burning excess fat is likely the primary reason many people take up some type of cardiovascular training. Over 50 per cent of the people who perform cardio in an attempt to burn fat are wasting their hours and hours of time! How? Most people are *not* performing the right 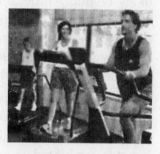 type of cardio workouts. Generally speaking (not including a 2 to 3 minute warm up and cool down) fat burning sessions should last no longer than 30 minutes. Further, to ensure that we are training effectively and remaining in our 'fat burning zone' we must monitor our heart rate. Our body works like a machine. If it is not provided with the necessary fuel it won't run efficiently. Therefore, unless we are at least at the low end of our training zone we are truly wasting our time. To find that low end number, the following equation needs to be performed:

220–Age–Resting Heart Rate (RHR) × .6 + RHR.

The result of the above is the minimum beats per minute that our heart needs to work to burn fat. A word of caution however. When our body runs out of fuel or in this case, available stored fat, it turns to other sources of energy to continue functioning. This process of diminishing returns occurs between 35 and 45 minutes in our target heart rate zone. As our body continues to burn through its fat stores, it begins to derive its energy from protein stores (lean muscle mass). Also if we train too hard, even within that half hour, we may still be burning only our muscle.

To avoid training too hard you must limit the high end of your training zone to 15 per cent of you *maximum* heart rate. Therefore, 220–Age–Resting Heart Rate (RHR) × .75 + RHR.

If you do not hit your target heart rate range, you will likely be doing little to help improve your heart or shed that fat. You should stay within you target heart rate range and never exceed your maximum heart rate. This will keep you from overstressing your cardiovascular system while giving you the benefits you are looking far.

Doing exercises is one thing and doing the correct exercises, the correct way, in the correct numbers, with the proper target set in the mind is another thing. Always follow the latter and benefits are bound to come.

9

Exercise Benefits

Losing weight is as easy as burning more calories than we take in. However, we all know that while it may be easy theoretically, losing weight in practice is hard and frustrating. The largest amount of calorie burning comes from our basic metabolism. Our basic metabolism (B M R) is made up of all the chemical processes that help make energy for us to do our everyday activities. Basic metabolism can burn quite a few calories.

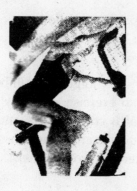 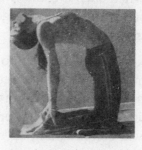

For example, a 60 kg woman may burn about 1,500 calories/day; a 80 kg man may burn about 2,000 calories/day, just through their basic metabolism. Therefore, in most cases if this woman ate less than 1,500 calories per day and the man ate less than 2,000 calories per day, they should lose weight. If exercise or other activities are added into a person's day he will burn more calories and if he keeps his nutrition the same, he should lose more weight. As a rule of thumb, for each mile he walks or runs he will burn 100 calories!

Therefore, he can see that walking or running for 20 to 30 minutes per day will help him burn another 200-500 calories per day. That may not sound like much, but if he just burns 200 extra calories per day he will lose 1 kg a month or 12 kgs in a year! If he combines exercise and simple changes in his nutrition he could easily lose more weight faster. You should keep in mind three important points while taking up any exercise regimen.

1. You must do things that you will be able to stick with.

2. It does not do any good to you to work hard to lose weight only to put it back on later. That's why many diets do not work—they are not changes that you can stick to. The rule is just to concentrate on simple and easy changes. Changes that you can stick to that will make sense for your lifestyle.

3. When such a concept is adopted and followed you find that with simple changes you will be able to lose weight and keep it off.

Exercise benefits are too many. But to get the full benefits you must know the correct way to exercise and how not to overdo it. Fitness experts, health consultants and gym instructors can give proper instruction and guidelines to be followed before taking up any exercise programme!

10
Lifting Weights: Facts

Every ten years past the age of thirty our body loses approximately ten per cent of muscle mass. Muscle requires calories and energy to exist. The less muscle one has, the fewer calories he will burn. Even if he eats the way he has always done without any changes, as he gets older if he doesn't lift weights, he will gain weight.

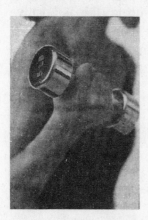

Muscle loss also accounts for poor balance and promotes injury due to falls, especially in older, frail adults. Muscle tone and flexibility contribute to good posture and can help prevent osteoporosis and lower back problems. In sports, the stronger athlete is the better athlete. Skill and timing may be crucial but strong muscles will help him make up what he lacks. *Muscular fitness* is a necessity, not a luxury, as one grows older.

Weight-bearing exercise builds sturdier bones. This is of particular importance to women who may be prone to osteoporosis due to decreasing estrogen levels during menopause on a genetic predisposition. Strength training is therefore important for preventing the muscle loss that normally accompanies the aging process. A common misconception is that as one gets older, it is normal to stop being active and to start using ambulatory aides like canes and wheel chairs. Many people think that they have no choice. They think it is normal.

But this couldn't be far from the truth. There is absolutely no reason why all of us can't be physically, mentally, and socially active, living a healthy vibrant life until the very day we die. The reason many elderly people rely on ambulatory aides and become slower and fatter over the years is because their muscles are decreasing. So their physical performance and metabolism also decrease, becoming less efficient.

From the above discussion it is clear that as one grows older one must lift weights! This 'lifting weights' will help in preventing muscle mass and also control 'putting on weight' nature. The muscle built burns the calories and avoids the extra weight accumulating in the body. Added benefits include strong bones and better balance. In simple words, 'one weight' prevents the 'other weight', i.e., weightlifting (this is positive weight) prevents the unwanted weight gain (this is negative weight). Hence, the weight in weightlifting is good weight and the weight in weight gain is bad weight!

11

Maximum Results in Minimum Time!

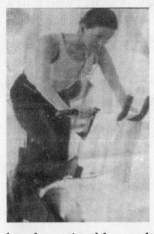

Most people who want to burn off some excess weight and tighten and tone their bodies simply don't have two hours each day to spend in the gym, doing the body building style work outs that most fitness experts recommend. Machine and free weight strength training are the best choice according to the health experts. But one need not have to make the gym one's home for many hours every day just to see slow, barely noticeable results.

It is not about training two hours a day or doing hours of high intensity weight training like a competitive body builder; or an hour and half of cardio a day like an endurance athlete, unless that's called for to reach a certain goal or unless that's what one enjoys. It is also not about lifting weights every day. One needs recovery time from intense terms of training.

What you need to do is some term of moderate exercise enough to break into a sweat, get your breathing heavy and bring your heart rate up—almost every day of the week, most

31

of the year. It could be the popular six-day programme alternating weights and cardio every other day with Sundays off. You must choose what you love to do—'Just do something every day' this must be the rule. You should include both strength training and aerobic training each week and do it on a regular schedule at the same time each day. Research says that for *fat loss*, five days a week for 30 minutes is much superior to three days weekly at 40 minutes even though the total weekly time of the three-day exercise is an hour longer. In order to keep the metabolic rate churning, *frequent exercise* is the key.

Daily exercise is essential to losing weight! Daily exercise is also very effective at changing a sluggish metabolism into a super-charged metabolism. Ultimately, the amount of exercise you need is the amount it takes to give you the results you want.

From the above discussion two important points stand out:

1. One need not be in a gym for hours, body building and intense weight training to stay trim and fit.

2. Consistent, regular, daily exercise is needed for weight loss.

12

Getting Rid of Stubborn Fat

Stubborn fat is the kind of flab that sticks to one in those hard-to-lose places. In men it is the annoying pockets right around the navel, lower abs, lower back and sides of the waist that make them want to leave their shirt out. In women, it is the grandmother arms, triceps flab. When she waves to someone those dreaded "saddlebags" dance! She also has to be bothered about those extra inches in the upper thigh, hips and butt area.

Fat storage patterns are genetic. The first place you stored fat is where you are genetically predisposed to deposit it. Then the person continues to deposit fat in those areas and spots, plus everywhere else on his body. Even the face and fingers— as the fat increases further. Once deposited he cannot selectively choose where he wants to withdraw the fat. He will lose fat all over the body and the first place he put it on will be the last place it comes off. That is why these fatty areas appear stubborn and why people continue to call it 'stubborn' fat. By the time someone loses enough fat overall to be down to the last localised 'pocket' (the first place he put it on first), he would have caused metabolic and hormonal damage from overly restrictive dieting. That is what makes the last fat harder to lose, not because the thigh/butt/tricep/ab fat cells themselves are most stubborn, but because the person is not burning as many calories as he used to. In fact, it can sometimes seem so hard to reduce those spots that many people become frustrated and resort to dangerous diet, drugs or liposuction.

Other people slave away day in and day out on the latest device. There is only one way to lose fat in the so-called "stubborn" areas, and that is with the correct combination of:

proper diet + aerobic exercise + weight training.

When such combination is followed consistently and judiciously a person will find to his astonishment that the stubborn, adamant fat begins to disappear and a trim and slim, fit body materialises to his satisfaction and happiness.

13

Flatten Your Stomach

Looking and feeling good are reasons enough for holding one's waistline. But beyond aesthetic and psychological factors there are some sound health reasons why strong, well-toned abdominal muscles are important.

They support and protect some of the most vital organs and increase their efficiency. Our abdomino pelvic cavity contains the liver, gall bladder, stomach, intestines, pancreas, spleen, bladder and kidneys. Strong abdominal muscles support the membranes that keep these organs in place and enable them to function properly.

By giving proper support to the lower spine, firm abdominal muscles help avoid or eliminate lowest back pain. They can help prevent or clear up some of the complications of constipation.

You, me or anybody can build and maintain a firm and flat stomach by adding a few abdomen strengthening exercises to our daily routine. These exercises are not intended as substitutes for but as supplements to diets or other exercises designed to reduce fat.

As with any exercise programme you must first consult a doctor. The exact amount of exercising you have to begin with depends on your age and physical condition. You must start slowly. These exercises should be approached gradually as some are simple and some rather difficult. Half the exercise can be tried with one repeat at first and then the other half repeated once. If there is a feeling of stiffness or soreness the next day, it means 'too much' was done. Gradually, you must reduce the number of exercises in one day's session and increase the repeats to a level that feels comfortable. Twelve repeats of eight exercises is quiet a good score. If you can't do them all, you can do those you can and need not worry about the rest. If a particular exercise seems too difficult or causes pain, stiffness or soreness it must *be left out*. After several months of conditioning, you must see whether you can add more exercises without strain; if not, it must be left out again!

Exercises must be done daily. Although any time that is convenient is fine, you are less apt to become a dropout if you do exercises first thing in the morning. Before you begin you must measure your girth at the level of your navel with your stomach relaxed. Then you must pull your stomach in as far as you can and measure it again. Both the measurements must be recorded. This must be done once a month on the same date and the recording noted. You will notice improved abdominal strength in a few weeks, but visible improvement may not be seen for a month or more. You must keep at it.

1. Lie on your back, arms stretched overhead against the floor, buttocks resting on the floor, knees drawn up close to your chest. Now extend one leg

Exercise 1

straight out, parallel to the floor, but not quite touching it. That knee must be drawn back close to the chest while extending the other leg straight out. Now the second knee must be drawn back, while again extending the first leg and you can just continue this bicycling movement through extensions of each leg.

2. We all have spent out entire life expanding our chest while inhaling and relaxing it (allowing it to become smaller) while exhaling. But it is possible to expand the chest after completely exhaling. To practise this, you have to inhale deeply and try to feel the way your chest expands. You must think only of expanding your chest and not of

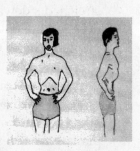

Exercise 2

pulling in the air. Just allow the air to come in as you expand your chest. You will find that you can expand your chest just as much as when the air does not rush into your lungs. Finally, you must exhale completely, hold the exhalation and expand your chest. If you do this correctly, you will see that your stomach will automatically pull in. Then you must try this exercise:

Stand with feet shoulder-width apart, hands on hips. Exhalation must be complete and forceful. Holding the exhalation, expand your chest as much as possible. The stomach must be pulled in tight for 6 seconds. Then relax to starting position.

3. Lie on your back, legs bent, with knees pointed towards the ceiling, feet flat on the floor, hands on the back of your head, fingers interlocked. Exhale as you lift up, and place head between your knees. Inhale as you lower back to the

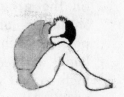

Exercise 3

starting position. It may help to keep your feet in place if you stick them under some heavy furniture, such as a dressing table.

4. Stand with feet comfortably more than shoulder width apart, arms stretched sideward and parallel to the floor, with elbows straight. Keep feet planted firmly; then slowly twist the trunk as far to the right as possible. Then stretch, pulling right arm back and left arm around to the right. Snap back to starting position and place hands on hips. The exercise must be repeated, twisting to the left.

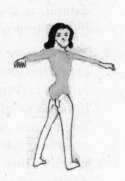

Exercise 4

5. Stand with feet straddled as wide as comfortable, arms overhead, elbows straight, hands shoulder width apart. Rapidly swing the upper body forward and down, while bending your knees. Reach back through legs and touch the ground as far back as possible. The upper body must be swung back to the starting position.

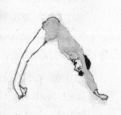

Exercise 5

6. Lie on stomach, hands above hips and close to sides, elbows pointed at the ceiling, palms on the floor with fingers pointed towards shoulders. Keep feet on the ground, and raise head, shoulders and chest as high as possible, arching the back. Keeping hands and feet in place, lift the rear high so that your body becomes an upside down V. Bearing your weight on hands and feet, knees and elbows straight, pull in stomach and tighten it. This position must be held for 6 seconds. Then lower the rear to the original arch, then back to the starting position.

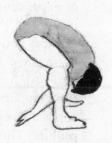

Exercise 6

7. Sit with legs bent, knees pointed towards ceiling, feet flat on the floor (preferably supported as in exercise 3), hands on the back of head, fingers interlocked. Lean back until upper body is at a 45 degree angle, then twist completely left, then right; then return forward to the starting position. The exercise must be repeated, twisting first to the right, then left.

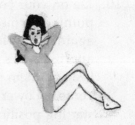

Exercise 7

8. Stand with feet shoulder-width apart, hands on hips. Reach over top of head with left hand, touching the right ear. Next bend sideward to the right, sliding right hand as far as possible down the right leg and stretching the left side as much as possible. Do not reach forward or backwards to slide right hand further down. Return to starting position, and repeat to the left.

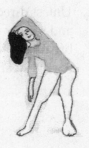

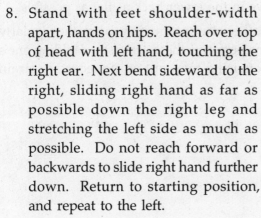

Exercise 8

9. Stand with feet shoulder width apart, arms at sides elbows straight. Lift right hip sidewards towards the right shoulder, allowing right foot to come off the ground. Do not move the right leg sidewards or think of lifting the right foot. Just allow it to come up. Lift the hip high, trying to touch the hip to lowest rib. Return to the starting position and repeat on the same side before repeating on the left side.

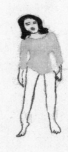

Exercise 9

10. Lie on your back, feet together, toes
pointed, arms stretched overhead
against the floor, shoulder-width
apart, elbows straight. Raise legs,
keeping them straight until they are
vertical. Lower the legs slowly to the
starting position.

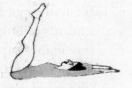

Exercise 10

Note: Since people respond in varying ways to any exercise
programme medical and physical fitness experts caution:

1. In doing exercise that involve the lower back—true of
   abdomen—strengthening exercise—it is very important
   to keep the curve in the lower back as flat as possible.

2. Unless directed otherwise one must try to breathe regularly
   and slowly as one performs these exercises. Holding one's
   breath while exercising may put an unnecessary strain
   on the heart.

14

Various Diets

Promoters of the popular low carbohydrate, high fat Atkins diet say that people should limit their intake of saturated fat by cutting back on Atkins staples such as meat, cheese, and butter. There have been criticism from scientists that Atkins could lead to heart disease and other health problems. There has been a revision of Atkins diet to tackle the above-mentioned criticisms. The revised Atkins diet suggests that only 20 per cent of a dieter's calories should come from saturated fat. Beef, pork, lamb, and butter were on the list of "foods you may eat liberally" in diet founder Dr Robert C. Atkin's book *Dr Atkin's New Diet Revolution*. While adopting Atkins diet one must keep the 'revised' diet instructions in mind.

A common doubt expressed to doctors by the patients is: can prescription drugs interfere with vitamin supplements? The answer is: Yes! Some prescription drugs can remove vitamins and minerals from our body or affect absorption ability. One can check with a *nutritionist* or naturopathic physician to learn whether one is at risk.

Rainbow Diet

The rainbow diet involves eating vegetables from each of the food colour groups to get a broader variety of important phyto nutrients.

Examples: Red tomatoes, purple grapes, orange, sweet potatoes, yellow corn, green spinach, white broccoli.

South Beach Diet

Invented by cardiologist, Dr. Arthur Agatston, this tells dieters that it strikes a balance between low carb and low fat. The diet is loosely founded on glycemic index of foods. The South Beach Diet runs in three phases:

Phase 1 sounds very much like Atkin's Diet with normal quantities of meats, olive oil, lots of vegetables, cheese, nuts, etc. No carbohydrates for the first 15 days—this means no bread, no pasta, no rice or wheat, no sugar, no sweets, no cookies, no pastries, no alcohol, and no fruit! This phase is high protein, high fat. The diet claims that one can lose about 4 to 6 kgs in that time. The minuses of phase 1:

a. Most of the initial weight loss is usually water.

b. A nutrition supplement might be required to make sure that the body doesn't get deficient.

c. A sudden decrease in carbohydrates, particularly sugar, alcohol and other high calorie foods, which are much a part of the Western diet, can, to some extent, explain the weight loss.

d. Piling on animal proteins and fats will only increase the risks of heart disease, cancer, etc.

e. This can become monotonous if followed regularly.

Phase I comes with a vegetarian option as well—meats are replaced with pulses, dals, soya foods.

Phase 2 reintroduces carbohydrate foods but rather slowly to prevent weight gain. Bread, pasta, rice, cereal, chocolate, wine and fruit are brought into this phase. This phase lasts till the target weight is reached, which could be a long time! Weight loss expected is up to 1 kg a week, which sounds reasonable. However, if one gets stuck at a particular weight, one needs to go back to phase 1 again!

Phase 2 might be more nutritionally balanced and requires patience to reach the target weight.

Phase 3 is called *Diet for Life* where normal foods are allowed in 'normal' quantities for maintenance of the lost weight. Yet, some foods that are higher on the glycemic index are not allowed in this phase also, and this is not based on fact. Changes have also been announced recently. Tomatoes, carrots and onions which were earlier restricted in the first two phases, are now allowed more freely.

GM Diet

Almost everyone who wants to lose weight has heard of General Motors Diet, commonly known as GM diet. It was originally developed for employees and dependents of General Motors, Inc. and was intended for their exclusive use in the 1980's. The GM diet makers also believed that it would improve attitudes and emotions because of its cleansing effects in the body. The seven-day plan is thought to burn more calories than the body receives. Theoretically, yes. But the human system is rather complicated.

The rules read thus: no alcohol, compulsorily 10 glasses of water per day.

1. all fruits except bananas on day one.
2. all vegetables on day two.
3. a mix of fruits and vegetables on day three.
4. bananas and milk on day four.
5. beef and tomatoes on day five.
6. beef and vegetables on day six.
7. brown rice, fruit juices and vegetables on day seven.

Beef has been replaced with rice in the Indian version. The diet would sound bizarre to any nutritionist! A repeat is advised for further weight loss. Pulses are disallowed because they are high in calories. Recipes have been made up revolving around the GM diet.

On the positive side, GM diet is good for a week if done once in a blue moon to cleanse the system. However, naturopathy medicine doesn't allow any kind of meat for cleansing the human system. Only those who can withstand the low energy intake should go for it. On the negative side, when on such a low energy diet the body tends to hold back the fat reserve and burns muscle for energy that is required for daily activity. The second and subsequent attempts at weight loss become more and more difficult because the basic rate at which the body burns calories (BMR) slows down. Following this diet repeatedly can deplete the body of energy and some important nutrients when needed. Unfortunately, we cannot supply nutrients in instalments on different days for the body because the functioning of all nutrients is interrelated. Many followers of GM diet have steadily gained back their weight.

We don't need Western diets to help us with weight loss. A sensible Indian meal pattern works very well for weight loss and good health.

Yoyo Dieting

Yo-yo dieting refers to repeated weight loss and weight gain. The syndrome begins when someone loses a noticeable amount of weight, usually on a restricted-calorie diet and then regains the weight. More often dieters regain all of the weight lost when returning to their normal eating habits. This may cause them to restrict calories again, lose more weight and begin the yo-yo dieting cycle again.

Diets suggesting too few calories can cause low blood sugar level and the symptoms that accompany hypoglycaemia: sluggishness, drowsiness, irritability, jitters and the more serious condition of fainting.

Dieters who have cycles of weight loss and weight gain get fatter each time they put the weight back on. During short-term dieting, if the dieter is not exercising, half or more of the weight loss may be due to a loss of muscle. This muscle loss can cause three problems. First, with less muscle, the dieter winds up thinner—but weaker. Second, since *muscle*, not fat burns calories, it is harder than ever before the dieter to maintain weight. Third, as weight is gained back it is mostly fat, since food alone, without exercise, will not build muscle.

By only restricting calorie intake, chronic dieters condition their bodies to survive on fewer calories, thereby putting themselves at greater risk for weight gain with the slightest increase in calorie intake. Exercise can help offset metabolic slowing by increasing lean body mass which means a person's body will burn more calories at rest. Sticking with one's exercise programme is crucial to maintaing one's optimum weight. It helps prevent the regaining of weight.

Yo-yo dieting can upset one's personality as well because it is disheartening to regain lost weight. It is better to lose weight more slowly and maintain the loss. In some circumstances yo-yo dieting can result in poor body image and a negative attitude towards food.

Yo-yo dieting has become a very hot and happening topic of discussion in health circles. Health experts, diet consultants, and nutrition experts are studying this phenomenon with more and more interest. A better understanding of this problem can shed more light on its preventive measures. Being aware of yo-yo dieting can help one avoid it, by self-discipline and control.

Common Doubts

A common doubts expressed to fitness experts is "Can I lose weight by exercise alone? A new study demonstrated that overweight people could prevent further weight gain by walking briskly for 30 minutes per day. Some even lost a few pounds, *all without dieting*; study participants who get no exercise gained 2 to 5 pounds.

Another common doubt in the minds of people is 'What is the average weight gain of a person without exercise?' Without exercising (certain statistics available for Americans) the average American gains about 1 pound of fat per year from age 25 to age 50.

15

Breakfast is Important

What is an Ideal Breakfast?

Most of the parents know that children who eat breakfast do better academically and have fewer behaviour struggles in school. But children however think and feel that skipping breakfast will help them lose weight or maintain an attractive weight. Just the opposite is true! Children who don't eat breafast tend to snack more, and they eat lunches and dinners that are higher in calories. It is important to make breakfast a priority, say health experts. Whatever be the excuse, kids need to eat breakfast. Skipping breakfast is a big problem. A lot of schools give mid-morning snacks because children skip breakfast. It helps their attention span.

There are plenty of options for a nourishing and low fat breakfast that can be made in spite of a tight schedule. Ideally, the first meal of the day should provide almost one-third of the nutrients the child needs until bed time. Protein, a carbohydrate and a fruit must be included as a rule. Scrambled eggs, cheese, yoghurt, drinks, peanut butter are all favourite protein foods among children.

Cereal is the obvious choice for carbohydrates. Children will benefit from a brand that has 10 gms or less of sugar and 2 or more gms of dietary fibre per serving. Fibre provides the "full" feeling, so the child does not feel hungry soon. Instant oatmeal or a cold oat or whole wheat cereal would be a good option.

Children can be given toasted frozen waffles with pureed fruit or light syrup or a toasted English muffin. It will be hard for the children to get the recommended two to four servings of fruit a day if they don't get a serving of fruit for breakfast. Something as simple as banana slices over a bowl of cereal or sliced strawberries in yoghurt can be prepared. The super-markets and food shops of today are selling so many varieties of such foods that one doesn't have to prepare anything! Just pick and choose the food you want from the shop. Yes! There is one big problem—the choice! It becomes a real problem to choose and pick from such a wide and extensive choice of products! All nutritious (tasty), delicious and highly desirable—to both the parents and their children!

A common doubt is

Can I lose weight by skipping breakfast? A recent study revealed that 80 per cent of those who lost at least 30 pounds and kept it off for a year or more ate breakfast. So the inference is

—eat a balanced breakfast.

—don't skip a breakfast.

—the breakfast must be appropriate in quantity and quality.

Fruit juice is fine but recommendation is 4 to 8 ounces serving. Milk must be encouraged before juice is served. The protein content of milk is a very important point to be considered. Solid fruits are much better than juice as it is more filling. If time is the obstacle the table should be all set in the night before, with everyone's cereal boxes and bowls. And when there is real rush, one can just pack a breakfast sandwich, such as peanut butter and apple slices, that the child can eat on the way to school.

Though the idea may sound bad, one can wake up earlier and fit breakfast into the routine. One has to take 10 or 15 minutes to eat a decent breakfast. It the parents sit down to breakfast, children also follow them. This 'role model' idea is a good concept. In some families breakfast is the only meal people have together to connect.

Cheddar cheese, whole wheat bread, scrambled eggs, peanut butter sandwiches, banana/apple slices, yoghurt, strawberries, high fibre breakfast cereals, almonds—all these can be mixed and matched, and interesting breakfast items can be made. With microwave, grill, toaster all at hand nothing is really a big deal.

Nobody really disputes the importance of a good breakfast. Certain fundamental mistakes have however been made in this important meal of the day under the false assumption that it is good. Let us consider some important points in regard to this context.

Breakfast outside United States is typically much smaller and healthier than what Americans consume. In the Mediterranean and north Africa, for example, breakfast is likely to include goat cheese, bread, olives, fava beans. In Malaysia, India, etc. rice is often on the menu.

Our ancestors were forced to rise early and perform hard manual labour. They needed a calorie intensive meal in the morning just to get through the day. But in the more sedentary culture that exists today many of us eat breakfasts that are far too caloric than we need, especially if we frequent restaurants that boast hearty breakfasts menus. Some of these breakfasts can supply a whole day's worth of calories, fat, sodium and cholesterol but very few of the other nutrients that the body needs to stay healthy.

A good morning meal should provide energy that burns steadily all morning long. For these who think that skipping breakfast is the answer to weight control medical researches point out that this is counter-productive. Study after study shows that people who skip breakfast take in more calories later in the day than people who eat three evenly spaced meals. The following suggestions will help in overcoming obstacles to a healthier breakfast:

1. If a person is just not hungry in the morning, he must start small. Drinking a glass of juice or eating a handful. Later on, when he really feels hungry, he can take some low-fat yoghurt, a wholegrain sandwich, or a slice of low-fat cheese.

2. If there is no time for breakfast he must keep some quick-to-prepare foods on hand like wholegrain cereal, non-fat milk, instant hot cereal packets or low-fat yoghurt. One can prepare and package foods the night before. For example, cut up fresh fruit, or spread peanut butter on whole wheat bread and pack it to go for the morning. One can also spend a little time during the weekend preparing foods for the week. Good diet is often just a function of good planning.

3. Thinking must go beyond the box. What is wrong with a bowl of vegetable soup and some wheat crackers for breakfast? Leftovers can be just as good for breakfast as they would be for dinner.

Breakfast to be ideal must consist of one-third or less animal protein (preferably low fat) and two-thirds or more vegetables, fruits, wholegrains and beans.

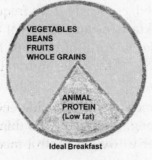

Ideal Breakfast

16

Eating Sensible Food

Green Leafy Vegetables

Green leafy vegetables are commonly called Greens. They have distinct flavours. Some are acidic, some sticky, and others bitter. Green leafy vegetables contain all important nutrients required for growth and maintenance of health and prevention of diseases.

1. Generally, green leafy vegetables have a high water content (85-95%) and a low fat content. Greens have a very low calorie content.

2. Green leafy vegetables are valued mainly for their high vitamin and mineral content.

3. Greens are a rich source of calcium, iron, beta carotene, vitamin C, riboflavin and folic acid.

4. The intensity of the green colour is an indirect indicator of the 'vitamin A' value of leaves. The dark green leafy vegetables are a rich source of beta carotene.

5. Greens contain complex carbohydrates such as cellulose, hemicellulose (fibre) which absorb water, increase the surface area of the food mass and thus help digestion and absorption of nutrients.

51

6. They help to ensure the smooth movement of food through the digestive tract.

7. The fibre present in greens helps to reduce blood cholesterol levels.

8. It is also helpful in preventing a sudden rise in blood sugar level which is particularly beneficial for diabeties.

Walnuts

Evidence has now come from researches that walnuts can reduce the risk of heart disease. Chopped or whole walnuts— whatever be the choice — eating 42 gms of it each day could help fight heart disease. Walnuts must be part of a low saturated fat and low cholesterol diet and not result in eating too many calories. The findings are only supportive and not conclusive.

Diet Eggs

An egg has a lot of Omega3 polyunsaturated fatty acids. It also has high 'Vitamin E' concentration. 'Omega-3' decreases cholesterol levels; cancers are prevented; doesn't favour atherosclerosis (fat plaques in artery walls). Omega3 also boosts resistance against diseases. 'VITE' is an antioxidant and has anti-aging properties too.

Soya, the complete plant protein, soyabean, belongs to the legume family and is a native of East Asia. It has been an important source of protein in the Eastern countries for thousands of years. Scientists and researchers concur that soya protein is complete. For many years we believed that complete protein (with all essential amino acids) came only from egg and milk. Therefore, egg or milk were pushed down everyone's throats, saying that they are the only foods that give all the essential AA's needed for the body and which the body cannot synthesise. Now research shows that soya protein is as good as milk and egg protein. Epidemiological studies indicate that incidence of chronic diseases like coronary artery disease is much lower in the Japanese population because they consume more than 50 gms of soyabean a day. There is an increasing evidence that consuming protein regularly may help to lower cholesterol by binding bile acids. The isoflavones (antioxidants) present in soya is believed to reduce cancer cell activity. Unlike animal protein, soya protein decreases calcium excretion from the body and therefore may help in controlling osteoporosis. Soyabean is high in fibre and has a low glycaemic index which helps in better control of blood sugar levels. Soya has more fat and protein compared to other pulses like bengal gram, black gram and green gram and has fewer carbohydrates than these pulses. Soya contains a good amount of vitamins, mineral and fibre. How to eat soyabeans? —is the main question. Here is a recipe one can try:

Soyabean Salad Ingredients

Soyabean soaked overnight	225 gms
Green gram sprouts	100 gms
Shredded spring onions	1/2 bunch
Olive oil	1 tablespoon
Lemon juice	2 tablespoons
Clove garlic crushed	1
Salt, pepper	to taste

Method: Drain soyabean. Add fresh water to cover and cook till soyabean is tender. Drain and rinse with cold water. Blend oil, lemon juice and garlic together and pour over warm beans. Toss and leave aside to cool. Mix with salt and pepper. Just before serving mix in the sprouts and spring onions. Serves 6; 160 calories per serve.

Drink like a Fish, Eat like an Elephant

"Drink like a fish but drink what the fish drinks"—this is a well-known saying. The following is an unknown truth: " Eat like an elephant but eat what the elephant eats." This means that one must eat the high fibre diet like the elephant does. High fibre diet is one single effective prescription for so many remedies ranging from simple constipation to major diseases like coronary heart disease, chronic constipation, colorectal cancer, hiatus hernia, gall and kidney stones, high cholesterol levels, all diseases related to high cholesterol levels and diabetes mellitus. Dietary fibre is that part of plant food which transverses the small intestine and is not digested by endogenous secretions. One of fibre's most important functions is to absorb water in the intestine to form a gel. It helps rapid passage of bowel contents. High carbohydrate high fibre diet causes slow release of sugar (carbohydrate) into the system and helps effective control of diabetic state. The fibre also helps in absorption, reabsorption, and metabolism of bile acids and cholesterol which are implicated in the pathogenesis of coronary heart disease and gall stones.

The richest sources of fibre food come from minimally processed cereals like rice, wheat, maize, ragi, etc.; legumes like beans, millets; root vegetables like carrots, turnips, leafy vegetables and fruits. "Retain the fibre in your food" is the doctor's advise to everyone. The following suggestions help in this.

1. Cereals should be processed as minimally as possible.

2. Avoid sifting rice, wheat, ragi or maize flour while preparing dishes out of them.

3. Pulses can be cooked with the skin.

4. Have vegetable fibre food with each meal.

5. Certain fruits can be eaten with peel, like apple, mango, etc.

6. Drink minimum two glasses of water with each fibre meal and in total about eight glasses per day.

17

Diet Food

Diet Food

Nowadays refreshment bars are popular at gyms where members can sip carrot juice, enjoy whole wheat sandwiches or nibble on an energy bar after a strenuous workout. Health bars attached to gyms offer fresh juices like watermelon, orange and other seasonal fruits. Yoghurt smoothies are very popular among many gym members. Sandwiches and wheat crackers which carry labels indicating the number of calories per serving are also very popular. Low fat bread, banana, apple cakes are also available in many gyms.

Many of the gym members have tight work or parenting schedules and often need something light to eat while on the run. Most office canteens and regular hotels serve greasy food, so the refreshment bars offering diet foods have become very popular. Certain gyms which have a health centre attached to the gym offer only juice and protein drinks. Papaya, carrot, betroot, orange, mango juices and energy drinks are the choices offered. Banana juice is offered in some gyms for weight gain. Most of the refreshment centres in gyms aim at offering a low calorie fat-free food to its members. Some gyms employ dietitians who design diet foods for the gym members.

Weight gain and weight loss foods are designed by dietitians. Salads, fruit, sandwiches, protein shakes made of skimmed milk and dry fruit are offered in such gyms. Many gym goers find refreshment centres an ideal place as they offer workout diet food and a platform to relax before a hectic day begins.

Vegetarians have lower rates of cancer and heart disease. Many major diseases begin with inflammation. Fruits and vegetables contain salicylic acid and inflammation-fighting compounds found in aspirin. In one study the blood of vegetarians contained 12 times more salicylic acid than the blood of meat eaters. This can very well explain the lower incidence of cancers, heart diseases in vegetarians.

Energy supplement: chromium 120 mg daily; phosphorous 1000 mg daily and a dose of vitamin $B_1 \rightarrow 1.5$ mg. These three substances can help one pick up one's energy. Mineral supplements and vitamins should never be ignored. Though they are needed in small quantities one must take them regularly and all the supplements are available as tablets.

Many people want to know what is the best way to add fibre to their diet? Very simple. One must always add fibres slowly in 5 gram increments for five weeks. If the person is tolerating it well, he can continue until he reaches a level of 25 to 35 gms.

A common doubt among women is: what cooking method is the least damaging? In a study using broccoli, microwaving zapped away 97 per cent of the flavinoids and antioxidants. Conventional boiling killed 66 per cent , high pressure boiling killed 47 per cent. Nutrient loss was only 10 per cent when the broccoli was steamed. So the present advice is 'buy a steamer and start steaming the veggies'. This is the least damaging of all the cooking methods.

Another common doubt needing clarification is regarding the healthiest rice of the 1,200 varieties of rice including

Jasmine and Basmati. Brown rice has the best nutrient profile because the Bran Jacket remains intact. The fibre, calcium, phosphorous, B_1 and niacin haven't been stripped away in processing as they have been with white rice.

Hidden sugar or added sugar: Every day the average person eats at least 4-6 teaspoons of added sugar. This is yet another reason to avoid processed foods.

Post-menopausal women can benefit from having 5-6 meals (small ones) per day, which helps balance blood sugar. After menopause slight diet modifications are essential. A woman must include more fresh fruits, vegetables, wholegrains. Regular exercise will also be beneficial to digestion.

A healthy alternative to salty white flour crackers is crisp rye bread. Many varieties are made with 100 per cent whole rye flour. Of course one needs to check the label to be sure.

Grape juice, papaya and pomegranate juices are very high in antioxidant compounds. But grape juice is the one with most antioxidant power. Medical experts recommend this as the best source for antioxidants.

Recent reseach says regular black tea is healthy. Black tea contains quarcetin, a compound that helps prevent blood clots, the triggers of heart attacks. When one plans a diet such points should be kept in mind. The diet must be balanced, nutritious, safe and must offer benefits as mentioned above. This becomes a complete diet.

To lower the risk of breast cancer, researchers suggest eating grapefruit regularly. Grapefruit contains the antioxidant compounds Naringin and Limonid. Naringin is found only in grapefruit. In lab studies, Naringin stopped the growth of breast cancer cells.

Research studies shows that those who ate authentic wholegrain rye bread reduced their levels of colon cancer promoting bile acid by 26 per cent.

A common question asked to the nutrition experts is: what is the best way to take calcium? Calcium doesn't absorb well when taken in large amounts at one time. If a person gets a lot of calcium at breakfast, he should take his calcium supplement at another meal.

One 12 ounce can of cola contains 10 teaspoons of sugar. Sodas and sweetened juices are the primary reason that the average teenager consumes three times their weight in sugar each year.

For healthier pizza one must order with double the tomato sauce and half the cheese. Lycopene rich tomato sauce is linked to reducing cancer risk. Half the cheese will lower one's consumption of saturated fat.

What kind of diet can minimise risk of stroke? Doctors recommend two ideas:

1. Eating fresh fruits and vegetables daily.

2. Eating bananas regularly. The equation for this concept is bananas = potassium = lower stroke risk.

A Practical Approach to Diet and Exercise

Anything done with conscious efforts, after reading health journals, listening to diet experts, etc., sometimes becomes a boring concept. Anything done with too much planning and thinking can become monotonous. This section discusses some practical simple suggestions regarding diet and exercise.

1. Participating in active sports can keep one fit.

2. Instead of making fitness a criteria, many persons unconsciously reap the benefits of health and well-being by simply leading a physically active life.

3. Restriction of 'triplets'—'sugar-chocolate-fatty foods' (of course keep in mind the latest reports on benefits of chocolates).

4. Any workout or sports must be done to develop stamina, strength and endurance.

5. Eat right and look fit (also feel fit).

6. Regular workouts indulging cardio, weights, etc., are fine. But playing cricket, half court basketball once a week, jogging for an hour three times a week are also equally benefiting (also more simple and practical).

7. One can wear clothes that fit well, deliberately to know when one puts on weight!

8. One can stick to seasonal fruits and fruit juices in the mornings. Lunch must be planned primarily with brown rice and steamed veggies. Dinner can be either fish or chicken. Never combine meats.

9. Some individuals let themselves go once a week. They forego their strict diet once a week and indulge in heavy meals, rich foods, mixed meats but the rest of the days they are on strict diets and regular workouts! But this 'one day indulgence' cannot be fine with everybody. Overweight individuals and ideal weight individuals must know their limitations. Nothing can be generalised and exceptions don't prove the rule.

10. There is no age limit to becoming fit. The Hollywood actor Sylvester Stallon started getting leaner after 50!

11. A trainer can chart out a personalised programme. Nobody should blindly copy or follow others in diet and exercise. Follow the principle of 'eat breakfast like a king, lunch like a prince and have dinner like a pauper'.

12. One must develop the right eating habits. Cooking must preferably be done in olive oil; less oil be used; veggies must never be overcooked; brown rice must be had instead of white rice; plenty of water must be taken and one must avoid mixing meats.

The Right Approach

One must identify the reason for depression. Find an outlet by putting the feelings into words either in a journal or by talking with a friend.

Emotional Eating: How to Tackle It

Certain people begin to eat when they are anxious, frustrated, bored, angry, sad, lonely or even when they want to celebrate something. During these emotional eating episodes the foods chosen are fatty, salty, sweet and/or high in calories.

How can one stop these emotional binges? This is a very unhealthy cycle and needs proper tackling. The first step is awareness. One of the best tools to help one gain awareness about one's eating patterns is to keep a food diary.

In addition to when and what a person eats, record of how he is emotionally feeling when he eats must also be made in the diary. Once a person consciously begins distinguishing *physical hunger* from *emotional hunger* he will need techniques to help him deal with his emotions. 'Sort out your feelings', recommend doctors. Instead of munching on a bag of chips without thought, he must take some time out to sort through his feelings.

1. **Stress**: He should visualise himself in a calm relaxing place while taking in slow, deep breaths.

2. **Boredom**: Almost everyone experiences this emotion at one time or another. One must select any activity or engage in some physical activity.

3. **Loneliness**: One must get together with, call or write to a relative or friend, volunteer some of one's time, join an organisation or get involved in one's community.

4. **Depression/sadness**: One must try to identify the reason for one's depression. Once one identifies it, one must try putting one's feelings into words either in a journal or by talking with a friend.

5. **Anger**: A person must take some time out and calm himself down by using relaxation techniques or going for a walk.

6. **Anxiety**: First the cause of anxiety must be found by the person himself. If it is caused by coffee or something that he has taken internally, he must try to find a way to correct the situation from happening again.

7. **Tiredness**: The person concerned must take a short nap or get some exercise.

8. **Celebration**: By all means he should celebrate! Celebration must include getting together with friends, going to a movie, buying something that he has been wanting or going for nice dancing. He can use his imagination. A celebration doesn't mean he must include food—and eat...eat...and eat! Or drink ... drink ... and drink!

18

Drugs and Obesity

Obesity is discouraged by modern society for social as well as medical reasons. The incidence of diabetes mellitus, hypertension, angina pectoris and myocardial infarction is higher among obese individuals.

Except for certain endocrine disturbances like cushings syndrome the etiology of obesity is not well understood. No intrinsic metabolic or biochemical abnormality has been identified in obese individuals. Recent research has been able to state that the fat cells of the obese are large (hypertrophic type of obesity). Some medical experts do not approve of this classification.

Although feeding and satiety centres have been identified in the hypothalamus of animals the role of the hypothalamus in the genesis of human obesity is not yet clear. Usually the obese are physically less active than the slim ones. Many obese individuals show psychological disturbances and a compulsive desire to eat, though such individuals may not derive satisfaction from the act of eating. In an obese individual if an organic cause is present it should be treated appropriately. Obesity due to endocrine disturbances falls in this category.

Commonly, obesity is due to excessive eating and lack of adequate exercise and not due to 'glands'. The patient must be made to appreciate this at the beginning of the treatment and must be explained clearly that diet is the mainstay of the treatment of obesity. For successful result the patient must be adequately motivated by the concept of positive health. It must also be emphasised that dietary treatment of obesity really consists of life long reorientation of his eating habits (and often those of his family) and not merely of a course of dieting. Individuals who look upon dieting as a course of treatment are bound to regain the lost weight and ultimately resign themselves to a crippled life of obesity.

There are as many diets for obesity as there are physicians and like other fashions, each diet has had its vogue. It has however been convincingly shown that in the long run nothing about the diet matters except its caloric content. Hence the best diet is one which is low in caloric content (1,000 to 1,500 per day), contains all the essential nutrients, provides a variety and is simple for the patient to follow for long periods. It should also conform to the patient's pocket. Proprietary slimming foods are expensive and are an insult to the patient's intelligence, as most patients seem to believe that they can lose weight by consuming them in addition to their normal diet.

Prolonged fasting is a drastic measure to be used rarely, only in resistant cases and that too under close medical supervision. The age-old Indian religious custom of fasting on certain days of the month has, however, most to recommend it, as it can help to keep good health. If the patient realises the importance of dieting and exercise and if he has the necessary will, then in most of the cases the treatment of obesity is not difficult and can easily be carried out at home without the help of obesity clinics and health clubs. The results of therapy are likely to be more satisfactory in the hypertrophic than in the hyperplastic type of obesity. The patient should be told at the onset of therapy that an average weekly loss of only 0.5 kg is excellent and would result in annual loss of about 25 kg.

Sometimes even with the best motivation drastic reduction in the customary food intake is initially a trying experience. In such cases appetite suppressants may help the patient to adjust himself to his prescribed diet. It must be emphasised, however, that these drugs only supplement and are not a substitute for the dietary restrictions; in fact, by themselves they are valueless in the therapy of obesity nor can they be recommended for prolonged use.

Anorexiants can be classified as:

1. Amphetamine and related compounds.
2. Bulk anovexiants.
3. Miscellaneous drugs.

Amphetamine and Related Compounds

Although their anorexiant effect appear to be related to the stimulation of the hypothalamus the exact mechanism of appetite suppression by these drugs is not known. These drugs may cause excitement, agitation, insomnia and sometimes psychotic reactions with hallucinations. Their major drawback is the development of tolerance to the anorexiant effect and later drug dependence. Withdrawal of these compounds after prolonged medication may cause drowsiness, sleep, tremors, fatigue and muscular weakness. These drugs are contraindicated in the presence of hypertension, hyperthyroidism and cardiovascular disease. The racemic form of amphetamine, because of its pronounce cardiovascular actions, is no more recommended in the treatment of obesity. The impounds employed are:

i. *Dextro amphetamine sulfate (Dexedrine)*. This drug has predominant central actions and weak peripheral actions. Dosage given is 2.5 to 5 mg. The drug should be administered only during the day, the last dose being given before 6 p.m. The drug, however has been extensively abused and should not be prescribed.

ii. *Fenfluramine (PONDERAX).* This analogue of amphetamine is claimed to have no central nervous system stimulant action. Further, it has been claimed to possess various metabolic actions in addition to its anoretic action. It appears unlikely that the metabolic actions as distinct from the anorectic effect contributes to the weight loss induced by this drug. It is available as 20 and 60 mg tablets. It is used in the dose of 20 to 100 mg tablets daily without restriction of diet. Weight loss is slow and tolerance can develop. Adverse effects, though mild, can develop and includes drowsiness, diarrhoea, dry mouth, insomnia, dizziness and headache. Although the drug does not cause central stimulation, mental depression during fenfluramine therapy has been reported.

iii. *Other compounds.* These do not offer any remarkable advantage over the compounds mentioned previously. Examples are phenteramine, phendimetrazine, benzamphetamine, mazindol, diethylpropion, chlorphenteranine hydrochloride. Of these the first four are suspected to produce dependence and could be abused. Mazindol is chemically unrelated to amphetamine.

Bulk Anorexiants

Methylcellulose is non-digestible. When ingested it swells and adds to the bulk in the diet. Though it is used as an appetite satiation in the treatment of obesity, it has proved no more effective than the high residue low caloric diet for the obvious reason that an obese person is interested in eating good food and not something that would merely distend the stomach. Methylcellulose forms an important cheap constituent of many 'costly' commercial preparations advertised for the treatment of obesity.

Miscellaneous Drugs

Thyroid and related materials: Though frequently used in the treatment of obesity, thyroid medication is not useful except to correct any associated thyroid deficiency. This is so because the doses of thyroxin required to raise metabolic rate sufficiently produce intolerable adverse effects.

Biguanides: Biguanides have been reported to induce weight loss in some non-diabetic obese individuals. This effect may be due to their anorectic effect, a reduction in gastro-intestinal carbohydrate absorption, and marked reduction in fasting and post-prandial hyper-insulinism which so often accompanies obesity. They have been used especially in patients with a family history of diabetes mellitus.

Drugs Causing Weight Gain

1. *Synthetic:* Gluco corticoids like prednisone, prednisolone, triancinolone, paramethasone, dexamethasone, betamethasone, 6 methyl prednisolone all these referred to by common man as 'steroids' can cause weight gain, cushing habits on prolonged use.

2. *Oral contraceptives:* Using progestogenestrogen combination, like medroxy progesterone acetate, can cause weight gain. Cushingoid symptoms can occur with high dose therapy.

3. Danazol, a synthetic steroid with mild androgenic action, causes weight gain.

4. Anabolic steroids like oxymetholone, stanozobl, nondralone, ethyloestrenol are protein anabolic agents with low androgenic activity. These steroids cause increase in muscle mass, increased bone growth, water retention.

Sweeting agents are non-carbohydrate substance devoid of food value useful as sugar substitutes in diet and beverages. "Figure conscious" but "cannot-sacrifice-sweet-taste" individuals prefer these.

The compounds available are:

1. **Saccharin:** White crystalline powder with markedly sweetening properties. Continued use of saccharin in small amounts has been shown to be harmless. Saccharin tablet contains 12 mg of saccharin.

    1 tablet is approximately equivalent to 1 teaspoonful of sugar (7.5 gm sucrose).

2. **Sodium cyclamate:** This is 30 times more sweeting than sucrose. It has been used as a good food additive for the last 30 years without apparent ill effects. But certain controversies regarding its cancer-causing nature needs clarification.

3. **Aspartame:** This is a dipeptide formed by a synthetic combination of two natural amino acids, L-aspartic acid and the methyl ester of phenyl-alanine. It yields 4 kcal/g but is 200 times sweeter than sucrose. It does not make significant contribution to calorie intake.

19

Surgery for Obesity

Controlling Obesity through Surgery

Obesity is a problem that modern woman and man have been trying to combat. Obesity predisposes a person to heart diseases, lung infections, gall bladder disease, diabetes and disease of the joints. It also decreases efficiency.

Obesity occurs when the calorie intake exceeds the energy requirement of the body for physical activity and growth. As a result there is an accumulation of fat, which is stored as adipose tissue. The excessive adipose tissue may be distributed generally all over the body or it may be localised. The factors controlling the location of adipose tissue are not all known, but thyroid, adrenal and sex hormones play an important role. In women the excessive adipose tissue is distributed predominantly in the lower part of the trunk and extremities, while in men it is frequently more pronounced in the upper part of the trunk, often sparing the extremities. The most practical method to estimate the amount of body fat is by using the standard weight tables. A person is considered overweight if he exceeds the upper range of the ideal weight for his body frame. He is considered obese if his weight exceeds 9-10 kg of his ideal weight. Obesity can be caused by various diseases of the hypothalamus, and other endocrine diseases of the thyroid, adrenals, pancreas, gonads etc.

This chart compiled by LIC has found acceptance as standard weight chart all over India.

Height in Mtr	Men (kg)	Women (kg)	Maximum weights you may reach
1.523000	-	50.8-54.4	
1.545840	-	51.7-55.3	
1.57380	56.3-60.3	53.1-56.7	Up to the age
1.59920	57.6-61.7	54.4-58.1	of 30 years
1.62460	58.9-63.5	56.3-59.9	10% standard
1.65000	60.8-65.3	57.6-61.2	
1.67540	62.2-66.7	58.9-63.5	
1.70080	64.0-68.5	60.8-65.4	Between 30 & 35
1.76200	65.8-70.8	62.2-66.7	years. Standard
1.75160	67.6-72.6	64.0-68.5	is the optimum
1.77700	69.4-74.4	65.8-70.3	Weight.
1.80240	71.2-76.2	67.1-71.7	
1.82780	73.0-78.5	68.5-73.9	
1.85380	75.3-80.7	-	Above 35 years
1.87860	77.6-83.5	-	10% below
1.90400	79.8-85.9	-	standard.

However the most common cause is due to familial and cultural eating habits which are imbibed at an early age. Psychological factors also play an important role whereas a person uses food as a substitute for the satisfaction that ordinarily would be derived from other sources. Increased food intake could also be manifestation of depression, anxiety, and the resulting obesity may aggravate the tendency towards isolation or the ineffectiveness of performance.

Among the various modes used to combat obesity, diet and exercise are well known. Drugs have also been used. They are basically the drugs that depress appetite by inducing a sense of well being, but they have their own complications and side effects.

Liposuction

Liposuction is a procedure done under general anesthesia where a small incision (cut-1/2cm) is made on the skin and a long blunt hollow instrument is introduced in a plane under the skin and through the fat. Powerful suction is applied to the end of the hollow tube, which sucks out the fat. The tip of the instrument is blunt and on introduction pushes the blood vessels and nerves to the side. The instrument is like a large needle but with the opening at the side. Liposuction is done usually for those who have fat deposits which are localised. Such localised fat deposits are common in the abdomen, hips, around the outer side of thighs (riding breech or Jodhpur deformity), buttocks, knees, calves, chin, upper arm. All these areas are amenable to treatment with liposuction.

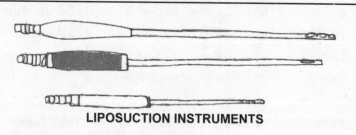

LIPOSUCTION INSTRUMENTS

What is <u>Lipo Augmentation</u>?

Transplanting excess fat from areas like height to skinny areas like face to make thin people look 'filled up', full and glowing.

What is Subemental <u>Lipectomy</u>?

Removing fat from the space between the chin and the neck. This place is usually the first to sag and drop. One can give a 'young look' by sucking the fat in this area and giving a taut firm look to this area (submittal area).

The blunt instrument or cannula is introduced in tunnel like fashion and the fat is sucked out. Up to 3 l of fat can be sucked out in one sitting leaving behind 1.50 cm of fat just under the skin (to give contour). After the surgery incisions are closed with one or two stitches. Compressive dressings are applied, which are removed at the end of 10 days to two weeks. Patients are advised to wear compressive garments for three months after surgery.

Liposuction is done ideally in a person between 20 and 50 years because it makes use of the inherent property of the skin to shrink when fat is removed from under it. After 50, the skin tends to lose the elasticity and the person may require an additional procedure. Those with not so ideal skin or who have plenty of redundant skin or if such redundancy is expected after liposuction, an additional dermolipectomy procedure, i.e, removal of fat and skin, is performed. This procedure leaves a scar somewhat similar to a transverse lower abdominal scar of a caesarian section. If the person already has such a scar, the fat and skin removal can be performed without giving the patient an additional scar. The number of fat cells in an adult remains constant. When one puts on weight, it is the size of the cell which increases and not their number (hypertrophy occurs, not hyperplasia). By removing X number of cells from an area, we are virtually ensuring that fat does not accumulate locally in the area again. This phenomenon is seen in practice. And those who continue to put on weight do so uniformly and not locally.

A phenomenon has been observed where a person who has undergone liposuction, especially of the outer side of the thigh, continues to lose weight — often a lot of weight — after the operation.

Complications of liposuction are mostly preventable. The risk of general anesthesia is always there. Infection and haematoma (collection of blood) are avoidable. Locally skin bruising and discolorations may occur but normally disappear in 10 to 15 days.

Morbid Obesity

Morbid obesity is a situation where a person is more than twice the normal weight for height. The death rate among these individuals is 12 times more than an obese person of the same age and sex. Severe obesity can predispose a person to a variety of serious disorders ranging from coronary artery disease, hypertension, diabetes mellitus, to marked ostoearthritis of the weight-bearing joints, respiratory distress, gall bladder disease and psychological incapacity. Frequently minor or standard operative procedures are major endeavours because of the anesthetics and preoperative problems directly related to obesity. Surgery for such morbid obesity has evolved over the years. Procedures short circuiting the gastro-intestinal tract so that food can be short-circuited to the large intestine before absorption can take place had so many disadvantages that it has been all but abandoned. Procedures which cause mechanical restriction like making the stomach smaller either by stapling or stitching it up or by introducing a balloon into it via an endoscope have become popular. These do not cause any metabolic disturbance by interfering with food absorption or digestion. The patient will lose a considerable amount of weight after these procedures. About a year later the redundant skin and fat is removed. Surgery is usually resorted to if other methods to combat obesity have failed.

Lap Band Surgery

A 'keyhole' type of stomach surgery called the Lap Band procedure provides good weight loss and markedly reduces obesity-related illness. Investigators also found that the procedure was safe enough to perform on an outpatient basis. The lap band is an inflatable silicone band placed around the portion of the stomach to limit the amount a patient can eat and slow the emptying of food into the stomach and intestine.

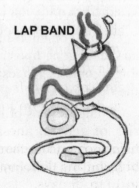

LAP BAND

The various good news about such surgical procedures are a welcome news as most of the obesity treating doctors feel that the only way to manage severe obesity long-term is surgery. The lap band procedure costs about one-third that of conventional stomach bypass surgery and poses far less risk of complications. The technique is also reversible.

In America lap band surgeries are being performed in large numbers. Out of 925 obese patients who got this surgery done between years 2001 and 2004 only 30 patients developed a post-operative blockage, all the others went home the same day of the surgery and only one required readmission after surgery. During one year of follow-up patients lost approximately 42 per cent of their excess weight.

Doctors of foreign countries where health insurance is a big issue feel that, even though surgery to treat severe obesity dramatically reduces health care costs over the long run, insurance companies are still reluctant to reimburse for these procedures.

The lap band procedure has become a popular topic of discussion is Western countries. They are being performed with increasing frequency. The operation also has beneficial effect on blood pressure, removed or improved diabetes in several patients and reduced acid flow out of the stomach in people who underwent such a surgery, report medical journals.

Surgeries for obesity have two different schools of thought. Some medical experts are against it and others have approved it as a suitable and best remedy for severe obesity requiring long-term solution. The Western countries have given a grand welcome to surgeries. In India, except for the affluent people, others don't opt for it. In India obesity surgeries are less popular. Fear of complications, high costs, etc., need clarification.

20

Diet and Exercise

Obesity is increasing in all the stratas of society but it is more common in the upper class or socially rich. Obesity cases can be spotted everywhere—in bus stops, shops, parties, schools and colleges. This only goes to show its prevalence. Obesity leads to disease and various other psychological problems. Overweight, obesity, being too fat all have become synonymous. As we have learnt earlier, obesity can cause various health problems like heart disease, stroke, arthritis and diabetes. Obesity also decreases a person's working capacity and efficiency. It limits his opportunities. The modern age with its various so-called 'developments' has made man lazy and paved the way to obesity.

Pot bellies, bulges, double chins, tyres on the back are all products of overeating, sedentary lifestyle and lack of exercise. A man stops growing when he reaches the age of 22 years. Some experts put this as 25. So there should be no increase in weight after 22 years. He should just maintain his weight at the ideal value (for his height).

The human body is made up of cells, fluid, bones and minerals. The fluid is divided into two categories: extracellular and intracellular fluid. Apart from all these components fat constitutes about 10 to 15 per cent of our body weight. Obesity is a condition in which fat gets deposited in excess in our body due to various causes.

Did You Know?

The average human body contains enough iron to make 3 inch nail, sulphur to kill all fleas on an average dog, carbon to make 900 pencils, potassium to fire a toy cannon, fat to make 7 bars of soap, phosphorous to make 2,200 match heads and water to fill a 10 gallon tank!!

There are also several other simple methods to assess obesity. Calipers (Harpenden) are available to pinch certain parts of body and determine the fat levels. Fat accumulates on the chin (double chin), neck, belly (pot or protruding belly). In the case of a woman, fat can accumulate in breasts, hips, buttocks. Self-examination can easily help in deciding whether there is excess fat or not. Any decrease in efficiency on capacity of doing a simple task, exertion and breathlessness on mild exertions—all indicate overweight. These things are self-explanatory.

Obesity leads to various ailments. The muscles of obese persons are weak and flabby. Arthritis is very common in obese persons. The weight bearing joints are under constant stress and strain due to excess weight of the body. Doctors often advice the arthritis patients to slim down. Blood vessels of obese persons get constricted due to excess cholesterol, which form plaques (atheromas). This leads to high blood pressure, stabbing pain in the chest (angina pectoris), heart attacks, strokes. The digestive system of obese persons is prone to diseases like diverticular pathologies. Gall stones may be formed due to excess cholesterol. Cancers, diabetes are all products of obesity. Obesity also creates problems during pregnancy. The various diseases and complications due to obesity shortens the lifespan of individuals and can lead to premature death. Mortality and morbidity are both to associated closely with obesity. An obese person not only suffers physical pains but also suffers psychological trauma. He feels inferior, and there may be psychological problems as he is often ridiculed and teased.

When a person gets into the process of reducing his overweight he benefits both physically and psychologically. He gains considerable control over diseases like strokes, diabetes, and hypertension; there are certain misconceptions associated with weight reduction. When an obese person resorts to diet + exercise regiment to reduce his weight, if he follows 'moderation' in his approach and is consistent in effort, he will definitely achieve a safe weight loss. There will be no sagging or flabbiness of skin. If he doesn't compromise on vitamins, nutrients and water there well be no problems. Hair loss, dry patchy skin, etc., may occur only if there are vitamin and hydration deficiencies.

We have already discussed the various causes of obesity, overeating, lack of exercise, sedentary lifestyle, genetic factors, endocrine (hormonal imbalances)—all constitute important causative factors of obesity. Among endocrinal causes we need to discuss certain syndromes. In syndromes we have a set of pathologies grouped in a very characteristic manner.

1. Cushing's Syndrome

This is due to excessive glucocorticoid hormones (cortical). This can also occur due to excessive corticosteroid administration. That is, both endogenous and exogenous cortisols can cause cushings. The clinical features are:

a. Wasting of tissues myopathy (weak muscles); thin skin, osteoporosis, purple abdominal striations.

b. Water retension oedema, 'moon face', high BP.

c. Obesity of trunk, head, neck (buffalo hump).

Apart from there they will be excessively prone to infection, poor wound healing, hirsuitism (hair growth in women).

2. Pickwickian Syndrome

This syndrome is caused by many factors; obesity is one of the causes. Enlarged tonsils, acromegaly, myxoedema are all other causes. What happens in this syndrome? During sleep there is collapse of pharyngeal walls leading to respiratory obstruction, sometimes for well over a minute. $\downarrow O_2$ and $\uparrow CO_2$ disturb sleep and there is daytime somnolence. Personality changes, intellectual deterioration, headaches, enuresis are all presenting features. One of the important aspects of treatment is to lose weight.

3. Laurence-Moon-Biedl Syndrome

There is polydaetyly (extra digits) retinitis pigmentos, cataract, microphthalmia, obesity, absent facial hair, hypogenitalism. This is a pituitary gland disorder. Also called Frohlichs syndrome or Adipose genital syndrome, some consider the fat boy of *Pickwick Papers* as an example of this syndrome. Others put him in the 'pickwickian' syndrome, i.e., obstructive sleep apnoea syndrome.

Thyroid and Weight Gain

A common question asked to doctors is, 'I can't seem to lose weight. Could it be my thyroid?'

The answer is: It is possible. But not likely. About 15 per cent of the female population has a thyroid problem. Of those, only 1 per cent can blame their thyroid for weight gain.

Thus we see in the above syndromes that either obesity is a cause or manifesting feature.

Here it will be of importance to learn about BMR (Basal Metabolic Rate). Metabolic rate is measured under so-called basal conditions (independent of exercise, extraneous factors). The metabolic rate is nothing but inherent activity of the tissues. The BMR implies the rate of energy utilisation in the body during absolute rest but while the person is awake. BMR is usually slow in a obese person's body and the excess food remains unburnt. This ends as fat. For all the overweight persons carbohydrates are the biggest problem. The excess unburnt carbohydrates also become fats (triglycerides).

Diet and exercise are the two important components involved in weight reduction. Diet must be designed in such a way that there is desired decrease in weight at the same time. The nutrition, vitamin and mineral status, and hydration are not compromised and are available in appropriate quantity and quality to the body. The basic priniciple involved in reducing the body

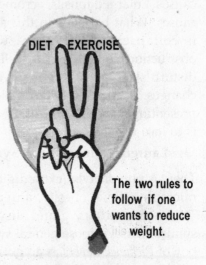

DIET   EXERCISE

The two rules to follow if one wants to reduce weight.

weight is, there should be more calories burnt and less calories eaten. The weight reduction diets keep the protein and fat consumed to approx. 40 to 60 gms and carbohydrate consumed maintained at 80 to 110 gms. Green leafy vegetables, fruits, sprouted pulses, are all consumed in adequate quantities to get the supply of vitamins, minerals, etc. Remember the dictum 'Too much of anything is bad'.

Exercise constitutes 'burn' parts of 'eat and burn'. Eat refers to proper diet and exercise aids in burning the calories to keep a balance. Otherwise there will be accumulation of extra calories as fat. Exercise regiments can be followed according to one's convenience, choice and requirement. Exercise not only reduces overweight, it also keeps the body fit and trim. This concept of 'body sculpture' is becoming popular both in foreign countries and India. We have already discussed about starvation. Some youngsters starve themselves to disease and debility. Fasting under medical supervision has been prescribed for certain unyielding types of obesity. Drugs and surgical techniques are also available for obesity treatment. Drugs working on the satiety centre of brain, drugs decreasing the levels of sugar in blood, diuretics are all being used. But generally using drugs to treat obesity is not very safe as there are many undesirable side effects. Liposuction as a cosmetic surgical procedure is known to all. Removing a portion of small intestines or whole of it (partial or total 'ectomys') to decrease the quantity of food absorbed is also done. The stomach is then connected to large intestines by passing small intestines. There are complications, etc., if the procedure is not done properly. Therefore, drugs, operation are extreme steps and are fit for only exceptional cases. They are best avoided in common obesity cases.

Diet + exercise form the main weight reducing strategy. Drugs, surgery, starving, etc., constitute extreme measures and all need medical advice and supervision. Ayurveda, unani, homeopathy, siddha, naturopathy, aromatherapy, herbal medicine, reflexology (grestalt therapy) magneto therapy, steam bath, yoga, body massage, psychiatric treatment with hypnosis, autosuggestion, etc., are all various fields and branches of medicine offering something or the other to reduce weight. Their benefits cannot be sidelined. These click for some obese cases and for others fail. Again if the patient or the person lacks will, motivation or effort nothing can work! A holistic approach including the various attributes of all the systems should be formulated. This can definitely work wonders. This should be in such a way that 'gains, positive attributes and excellent results' must be included from all systems and 'the side effects, negativities disadvantages' completely filtered and discarded. Hope something of this kind comes into the weight reduction regimens soon. It will be a boon to overweight obese persons and also to fitness-conscious individuals.

In reducing the overweight apart from the individual with the right attitude, motivation and will to reduce weight, a diet expert, a fitness expert, a doctor (if needed) all play an important role. When expert consultation is needed nobody should hesitate to take it. Books on such subjects can serve as guidelines; they should not be interpreted as Bibles and followed blindly. Merely resorting to something on 'own' without proper knowledge, skill or experience must be avoided.

Once a proper weight reducing strategy has been adopted and followed one must keep a check on the rate of weight reduced. Regular weight measurements help. Pregnant women, childhood obesity are all to be treated as special cases. The weight gain during the pregnancy period should be within ten kilos. The tendency to put on weight increases during pregnancy, as there is nutritious diet, unnecessary rest. The pregnant women must be cautious.

Childhood obesity is another important special case. Familial history, overfeeding, lazy nature, psychological trauma compensated with food, can all lead to childhood obesity, can create physical and mental problems to a child. 'Eat and burn' principle is to be followed for children. An ideal weight must be achieved with proper diet and physical activity not with starving the child.

21

Food Pyramid and Aerobics

We have all heard it time and again—eat only bananas for a week and you will lose 10 pounds, drink cabbage soup for a month and you will lose 5 pounds. The claims of fad diets are interesting to say the least. Do we ever bother to remember the food pyramid that we all studied in high school science? That is the basis of sensible nutrition.

At the base of the pyramid are carbohydrates—rice, wheat and bread. Next comes vegetables and fruits followed by meat, nuts, eggs and the milk group. Whether a person has six or 11 servings depends upon various factors. The only rule is to ensure that we get at least 1,200 calories a day. The sugar intake must be kept at a minimum and fat intake must be kept at 20 of the total calories.

When a person is on a calorie deprivation diet that does not include exercise he sheds weight extremely fast. This is because his body is burning protein for energy. Protein contains half the calories that fat does, so he burns double the amount to sustain the same levels of activity. Besides protein, muscle is four-fifths water. That reduces the quantity of energy derived by another one-fifth. Naturally the weighing scales seem so much friendlier! Unfortunately, by burning muscle protein the person concerned is lowering his basal metabolic rate as a result of which he will burn much less calories for the activities of daily living like sleeping or breathing. When he goes back to his normal eating pattern, the weight will come back with a vengeance, because his body is now much less adept at burning calories.

So, where lies the answer to the weight loss problem? It is simple really — a person has to raise his basal metabolic rate. Something that can be accomplished only by aerobic exercise— running, walking, dancing. They are the good guys that help one take the weight off and keep it off! To really see results he would need to exercise at least five days a week for 30 to 45 minutes at a fairly brisk pace. He should also get into some strength training. That way he will build lean muscle mass and every pound of muscle built burns 35 extra calories a day! He should not stop exercising once he has reached his target weight—he needs to keep on a maintenance schedule of about 30 minutes three to four times a week. There is nothing like exercise that can be stored in a bank! Just keep at it.

Don't Overstretch Fitness

Staying in shape is on everybody's agenda these days. But even as fitness conscious persons sweat it out in gyms some of them are ending up with complications, because they are over-exercising or doing it wrong.

Often ladies in their early 40s develop severe back pain within two or three months of joining some upmarket gym in their city. They have joined some weight loss programme. First everything goes well. Gymming and doing cardio-vascular exercises they often lose 4 kg or so in six weeks. But later they develop back trouble. When doctors treat such cases the patient herself comes out with the cause of her problem. "The place used to be so crowded, there was no personal supervision. The routine was almost the same for everybody and very rigorous. But it wasn't structured; we just used whatever machine was available. But after joining a less

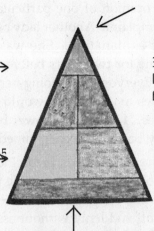

Fats & sweets: eat sparingly

Milk and cheese.:2-3 → servings

Meat and nuts: 2-3 servings (2-3 oz lean meat, poultry or fish=1 serving)

Fruit: 2-4 servings (1 ← piece of fresh fruit, ¾ cup of unsweetened fruit)

Vegetables: 3-5 servings (1/2 cup of cooked or raw vegetable=1 serving)

Bread and cereal: 6-11 servings (1 slice bread or ½ cup of rice=1 serving)

FOOD PYRAMID

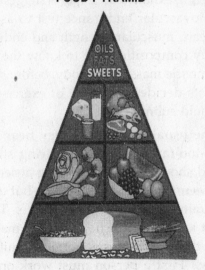

crowded gym I realised how important the sequence one follows is, was the opinion of one particular lady presenting the above typical complaint. Another lady of similar age group came with another explanation. She was going through a slimming programme for two years before realising the harm it was doing her. "Everyone was doing her own number. Of the several machines available we would rush and occupy the one that was free. I developed lower back pain, so did a lot of women in my batch" she complained.

Orthopaedic surgeons, sports medicine experts feel that the commonest problem with these people is not maintaining a graduated scale while starting an exercise. Mainly those in their 40s who start off suddenly without assessing how much they can take and those who get into unaccustomed activities without warming up or stretching end up with problems. Knowing one's capacity and understanding that not all exercises suit everybody is essential. Experienced fitness experts say, before any exercise, a fitness test has to be done. They should also work towards a goal instead of just exerting themselves and feeling exhausted. Experts suggest a series of tests like the cardiovascular endurance test to ascertain the condition of the heart, muscular strength and endurance test, flexibility test, body composition test to know the individual weight of fat and muscle mass in the body, before starting any routine. These tests decide what type of exercise and how much of it one should submit oneself to.

Doctors list the usual complaints they hear from such "fitness-stretched-too-far" cases as hamstring strain, groin strain, kneecap and shoulder injuries. Using a sleek machine at the gym might seem like the simplest thing but unless there is supervision by trained personnel it is not safe. Those using the machines must know the functions of each machine well. Haphazard use of these machines is not only fruitless, it can also hurt the body. First a person must work on his lower body which is relatively stronger, before the upper body consisting of smaller muscles. So he needs to follow a sequence while using the machines. Overloading the muscles is harmful. Certain persons who initially overwork and manage to lose weight get it all back as the routine becomes very tiresome and killing. Later they resort to a systemic routine in which there is no reduction in the weight, but inches are lost. For any physical activity to yield results it should be maintained throughout one's life. This can be through any enjoyable activity likes walking, jogging, swimming, stretching, etc.

But one message is loud and clear: don't stretch fitness too far. Don't overdo or do things haphazardly. It can prove dangerous.

22

Supplements and Exercises

Listening to a promotional lecture on a recently launched nutrition supplement, I wondered how many normal persons would begin to take them and how many of those people really needed them. Not only I but many of my friends asked an expert on nutrition the same questions. The expert said that misguided information about supplements is leading more people who need less or no supplements to take them. For example, recently a body builder's comment in a health programme on TV informed the viewers that one does not get adequate proteins by eating food and therefore one requires supplements!

The irony in our country is that those who really need supplements are the hungry or undernourished people who cannot afford to buy them. On the other hand, those who can afford to buy supplements and do take them regularly do not really need them because they can get adequate nutrients from natural foods if they balance their food intake well. Supplements are best utilised by patients in a clinical setup when properly prescribed by the dietitian.

Americans can easily buy 12 dangerous dietary supplements over the counter or over the internet! At least five of these supplements are banned in Asia, Europe, or

Canada. Imported supplements have arrived in plenty in India. The general public is not aware if these supplements are subject to safety checks or not. Sometimes the accompanying literature is not based on research, nor is the product time-tested. Only testimonials that cannot be proven true or false come along with supplements.

Most of these supplements are available through network marketing and not directly from the shop. Those who sell/ promote these supplements claim that the product helps to prevent a disease or disorder or promote healthy function.

Though many have long lists of ingredients and nutritional values printed on the labels, most consumers either do not read or don't understand the terms. Some studies show that a nutrient in excess can actually cause harm. The bottom line is that nothing can replace the goodness of natural foods and their nutrients. So the next time a supplement is pushed into your palms, think before buying it. One should ask for professional advice from a qualified nutritionist before buying it.

New Concepts in Exercises

1.Slow Burn

Wouldn't it be great if a person could trade his 45 minutes four-days-a-week workout for only 20 minutes once a week and reap greater benefits? It is possible, say advocates of the super slow workout, an increasingly popular twist on strength training. They claim that pumping iron at a snail's pace—10 seconds up and 10 seconds down—is so effective at building muscle and strength that it will help him speed his metabolism and lose more weight more quickly than a typical routine of aerobics and weightlifting. While other experts agree that strength training is important they say that aerobic activity is essential. Exercises such as running, jogging and biking have been found to reduce cholesterol and high BP and prevent heart disease. So 'super slow' is worth trying, say fitness experts but they also encourage aerobic training. Some research studies show that super slow produces 50 percent larger strength gain than regular weight training. But one must remember that it is extremely intense. In a programme of super slow workout out of the 147 participants only one or two continue doing it, says a study.

2.Water Aerobics

Across the length and breadth of America aquatic exercise is becoming increasingly popular as water has been found to be ideal for muscle toning, is soothing and increases stamina, strength, flexibility and endurance. It is well known that over-body weight is much less in water. Hence, when one stands in water at chest level his body is near weightless. The natural buoyancy of the water supports the body and relieves the stress on joints, tendons and ligaments. Water's gentle support enables easy and effortless movements. Many Americans with arthritis, old-age problems and post-operative recuperation, walk several times up and down the pool — usually such pools are 4 feet deep only at any point or all points or through its length and breadth. Such shallow pools are zones of wonderful therapeutic cure. In winter the swimming pool is heated and in summer it is kept coop. Many patients come to recover from injuries and after surgery also.

In water aerobics one needs to be in a swimming costume, and where required, to do the exercises standing in shallow water. There are exercises for the head, eyes and mouth, shoulder, inner and outer arm, thighs, legs, ankle, feet and fingers of the hand and toes, etc. In short, the exercises cover every part of the body from head to toe. Breathing exercises are also included. While land exercise aggravate orthopaedic problems water exercise can be done without undue stress and muscle weakness. The water's qualities are unique. Its elasticity adjusts to variations in force or speed of movement at different joint angles, thus providing a constantly changing resistance.

The fascinating and inviting qualities of water make the exercise smoother and more relaxing than land exercise. In water aquatics the combination of routine is limitless and there is something for everyone, even a non-swimmer. Just standing neck deep in water stimulates circulation; there is soothing effect on muscles; the heart in fact recovers more quickly from exertion because it is not working against the force of gravity. The water exercise includes 15 minutes of warming up and ends with 15 minutes of cooling down with a half hour of jogging and exercise in-between. Before undertaking any form of exercise one has to consult a doctor, and exercise intensity can be increased only gradually. In India too, water exercise needs to be popularised to promote muscle toning and other benefits.

Hospital Programmes

Hospitals too offer many diet and exercise programmes for both prevention and cure of overweight and obesity. Certain super speciality hospitals have custom-made programmes to suit individual needs of a patient. Some hospitals have created such programmes with the basic idea that most of the people don't even have enough time to take care of their body and health in this fast-paced competitive world. Health often takes a back seat as most people rush to meet deadlines and try to give more than their best to everything they do. Many people look into the mirror and wish they had more time to take care of their body. The hospital programmes have awareness seminars, which recommend three important points:

1. One way to keep oneself healthy is to fight fat.

2. This can be done with two important measures of eating nutritious food and work out.

3. State-of-the-art technology and innovative measures and techniques can make it possible to go beyond medicine and look at prevention.

Having recognised the role of diet in staying healthy, the focus is now on how to improve the lifestyle. Many these hospitals offer preventive health check-ups and tele medicine consultation and a host of other programmes focused at keeping people away from the hospital, creating a paradigm shift from illness to wellness. Certain hospitals setup wellness centres dedicated to fitness through adequate weight loss. 'Health and diet clinics' are the result of this endeavour. Such clinics offer a step-by-step scientific programme to combat weight. It starts with a health screening to check one's cholesterol levels, triglycerides (TGT), ECG, CSA (cardiac stress analysis Treadmill Test) and general physical condition.

The health screening will be followed by a session with a nutritionist who will recommend a diet plan that suits the person's personality.

Though it will be bases on the person's current dietary pattern it will be balanced so that the food he eats has a positive impact on his health and works along with his body's natural metabolism. Personalised diet programmes are available to fight cardiovascular diseases, hypertension, diabetes, obesity besides other health concerns of adolescents. The health programmes of certain hospitals also deliver diet at the doorsteps of persons concerned. Some hospitals serve a nice package of three balanced meals and two portions of snacks every day. The nutritionist will explain how the diet works on the person's body and the relationship between body fat and weight. So there is lot of interactive sessions and the nice communication skills of the nutrition expert pleases and convinces the person concerned beyond doubt. In India, the Apollo group of hospitals offer such programmes.

The programmes also stress on exercises. Since exercise is important in reducing weight, a physical training schedule based on every individual's body composition will be prepared and implemented. It will also take into account injury parameters and the health condition of the individual.

Fitness experts who specialise in strength cardiovascular system and Swiss ball training often chart out these programmes. The exercises are intended to increase the lean muscle mass and decrease body fat. Fitness testing includes cardiovascular fitness, strength flexibility, pelvic strength and stability and local muscle endurance. Special trainers will suppervise the entire fitness regime in these hospital-based programmes.

Most of the hospitals nowadays stress on preventive medicine. Obesity is no exception. Warning signals are looked for and treatment started as early as possible. This helps to avoid complications and makes the individual healthy. The hospitals often stress the implications of neglecting preventive health care. They are applicable to obesity also. The various implications are:

1. Complications in treatment
2. Disease beyond cure
3. Anxiety and fear
4. A worried and insecure family
5. Disturbed life and work schedule
6. Treatment hassles including expenses
7. Restricted life
8. Decreased productivity
9. Higher cost of medical care
10. Higher premium for medical insurance

This only goes to restore the old saying, 'Prevention is better than cure'.

From Illness to Wellness

Preventive health care is the tool that aims towards a shift from illness to wellness.

Illness	**Wellness**
Treat the illness.	Prevent the illness.
Incident driven.	Information driven.
Manage the disease.	Manage life.

The above concept applies to obesity and overweight also. It is better that we aim at preventing it rather than acquire it and try to cure it. Though hospitals offer both preventive and curative services we must always opt for the former. Hospitals also stress on this point.

23

Obesity and Vegetarianism

Chubby cheeks look cute only up to a certain age after which they are given the appropriate term 'face fat'. Not only do these layers of fat hide a person's cheekbones but also refuse to let him or her have a prominent jaw line. There are some simple exercises, which help a person get that fat off his face. If somebody expects quick results then he should prepare himself mentally as losing fat from the face is not as easy as putting it on.

Women especially have the tendency of having swollen faces. Water retention is a major cause behind that puffy face. Lack of proper diet, sleep or exercise is immediately reflected on a person's face.

Fat on the face can make the skin appear loose and saggy. To give it a toned look, one needs to do cardio exercises regularly. Walking or running on the treadmill, cycling and doing aerobic exercises are some of the best ways to get the appealing display of cheekbones. For best results two minutes of walking must be alternated with two minutes of running on the treadmill.

A high carbohydrate diet does more harm to a person's body. Not only does it result in weight gain but also makes a person feel lethargic and drowsy, bringing his activity levels down.

Double Chin

1. Throw your head backwards gently till you feel a strain on neck. Push your lower jaw forward and backward. This must be done whenever you are exercising or whenever you get the time, as many times as you can.

2. Check your posture while sitting or standing, as an improper posture can also be the reason behind a double chin.

If done regularly, these exercises which are simple to follow, can help in defining the frame of a person's face by making his cheekbones and jawline more prominent.

Vegetarianism—A Healthy Option

The word 'vegetarian' used to conjure up images of two extremes: holy people or the eccentrics, but not anymore. In fact, vegetarianism is fast gaining popularity with reasons ranging from religious and ethical beliefs to health or economic considerations.

Vegetarians eat most plant foods like vegetables, fruits, and grains although some do not include onions, garlic and chives. Generally there are three styles of vegetarianism based on other foods allowed as listed below:

1. Vegans are the strictest—they abstain from all animal foods, dairy products and eggs.

2. Lacto vegetarians consume dairy products.

3. Ovolacto vegetarians supplement with eggs and dairy products.

Prudent vegetarianism is highly beneficial. Studies show that vegetarians live longer, have lower blood pressure and cholesterol levels, register lower incidences of obesity, heart diseases, certain cancers, stroke and diabetes. These are not surprising as vegetarian diets contain less saturated fat, fewer calories, less sugar and more fibres.

Illustrious Personalities who were Vegetarians

Leonardo da Vinci, William Shakespeare, Benjamin Franklin, Leo Tolstoy, George Bernard Shaw, Henry David-Thoreau.

Leonardo da Vinci wrote condemning non-vegetarianism as "truly, man is the king of beasts, for his brutality exceeds theirs. We live by the death of others. We are burial places!"

Animal meat contains cholesterol, the main culprit that causes cardiac problems in human body. Barring a few products like coconut oil, most of the plant foods are free from cholesterol.

- Vegetarians have much lower cholesterol and LDL than the meat eaters.

- Vegetarianism is fast catching up in Western countries every year. In America one million people switch over to vegetarianism. In UK, according to the national vegetarianism society, 2000 people renounce non-vegetarianism every week!

Sprouts: Excellent nutrients

Sprouts contain reproductive power (embryo) that is of vital importance to human lives and their health. Germinated seeds enormously increase the nutritional value and digestibility. There is an amazing increase in nutrients in sprouted pulses as compared to their dried form. In the process of germination the vitamins, minerals and protein increase substantially with corresponding decrease in carbohydrate content. Cooked sprouts (steamed) are best to digest and avail maximum proteins.

Sprouts help in the growth of muscles and tissues of the body. They increase the resistance to diseases and play an important role in rejuvenation of cells.

Enticed by its goodness already? Now before anybody starts it is important to understand how to plan a well balanced vegetarian diet. Pregnant women, teenagers and young children should seek proper nutritional guidance before embarking on it.

The main concern in a vegetarian diet is protein. It is needed to build body tissues and consists of units called amino acids. Compared to animal protein like meat, plant foods generally lack certain amino acids. Hence, vegetarians, especially vegans, must eat a variety of plant proteins to get a complete set of amino acids. Soyabeans, a high quality protein, and its products like tofu and soya milk may feature frequently in vegetarian meals.

Vitamin B_{12} also needs monitoring for its deficiency causes anaemia. As animal foods are the only reliable sources of vitamin B_{12} substitutes like vitamin B_{12} enriched breakfast cereals are ideal. Furthermore, these cereals are also fortified with iron, much needed by younger female vegetarians. To optimise iron absorption, one must ensure an adequate supply of vitamin C in diet. Other good sources of iron are spinach, raisins, pulses. For non-dairy product eaters, calcium intake may be obtained from alternatives like sawi, spinach, and kailan. If seafood is omitted, zinc required for the immune system is obtainable from wholegrains, nuts and soyabeans.

When vegetarians are unsure of ingredients used in processed food or drinks, they may consult the manufacturer.

Vegetarianism is a healthy option provided careful meal planning is exercised where nutrients excluded from not eating animal foods are replaced. Indeed much discipline is needed to practise vegetarianism, especially in a predominantly meat-eating society.

Vegetarianism: Its Achievements

1. Overweight people who have tried a vegetarian diet have lost weight and kept is off.

2. Diabetics achieve normal blood sugar levels, reducing insulin requirements.

3. People with high BP, diminshed or eliminated their BP medications because BP was normalised.

4. People with high cholesterol showed lowered cholesterol levels.

5. In a majority of people with elevated homocyteine, levels were reduced, which is an improvement without the use of medication.

6. Overall endurance, strength, stamina, energy and sense of well-being achieved.

'**Cruciferous**' vegetables—cabbage, brussels sprouts, watercress, so named because of the cross shaped arrangement of their flower petals—and others are bursting with chemicals called Indoles that can block certain cancer-causing agents. These vegetables should be generously included in our diets as they offer a lot of benefits.

Slimming Tricks?

Designer diets, wacky tips, weight loss bestsellers—there have never been so many slimming tricks around. In the obsession to get thin many people can't even distinguish the food fad from foolish ideas. A weight-obsessed generation will do anything to get thin, and cashing in are a slew of new weight loss ideas and concepts—ranging from common sense tips to completely 'over the top' ideas.

1. Take, for instance, a recent study conducted by a clinic in Minnesota, which shows that fidgeting could keep a person thin and that those who have a hard time sitting still are the ones who will not gain weight. The study shows that the calories that people burn during everyday activities are very important for weight control. It

advocates moving around all the time, stretching, jumping off the couch to surf channels, fidgeting in a meeting—all to aid weight loss.

2. New weight loss books are also making headlines. The big newsmaker is entitled.

3. French women don't get fat: the secret of eating for pleasure touted as the best of the new crop of weight loss books, the basic message of the book is to eat only good food and relish every bite just as the French do.

4. Yet another fad doing the rounds is the coconut diet which pinpoints how people can utilise coconut oil to look and feel better and lose weight. It is believed that coconut oil contains ingredients that the body can metabolise quickly by converting fats to energy, instead of storing them.

Fads and concepts like these are very popular everywhere and everyone now obsessed with becoming thin. The fitness trends have a stressful impact on youngsters today. There is a 75 per cent increase in clients who want to get thinner in health centres today in the metro cities of India. Most of the youngsters are so obsessed with weight loss that they want to lose 10 kg in a month. This is a dangerous trend because ideally a person should lose only up to 4 kg a month.

People in the city are doing crazy things to lose weight, say health experts. Many youngsters follow fad diets like eating only cabbage or tomatoes or bananas daily. Taking pills and powders is another popular trend. Women go into severe depression if they even gain one kilo. Nutritionists believe that the obsession to lose weight is taking strange turns. Youngsters who are already thin feel they are fat. They set crazy targets for themselves, try diet after diet or go overboard with gaming or aerobics. Health experts categorically, no gadgets, no diets, no pills, no powders will help. Only balanced meals, regular exercise and elimination of fatty foods from the diet can make a person thin.

Food Addiction

People who say they are addicted to chocolate or pizza may not be exaggerating, say US based scientists. A brain scan study of normal hungry people showed their brains lit up when they saw and smelled their favourite foods in much the same way as the brains of cocaine addicts when they think about their next dose.

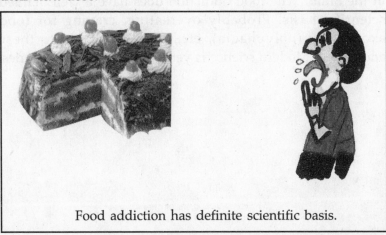

Food addiction has definite scientific basis.

Food presentation significantly increased metabolisms in the whole brain and these changes were the largest in superior temporal, anterior insular and orbits frontal articles (certain areas of brain). These areas are associated with addiction. For instance, the orbits frontal cortex has been seen to activate in cocaine users when they think about the drug. These results could explain the deleterious effects of constant exposure to food stimuli, such as advertising, candy machines, food channels and food displays in stores. A research study was taken up in America. Volunteers were asked to fast for just under a day and then underwent a PET scan, which measure brain metabolism. They were asked to describe their favourite foods and how they like to eat them while they were presented with some of those foods. A cotton swab impregnated with the food was placed in their tongues so they could taste it. The favourite food items most frequently selected by the subjects were bacon-egg-cheese sandwich, cinnamon bun, pizza, hamburger with cheese, fried chicken, lasagna, barbecue rib, ice-cream, brownie and chocolate cake.

This discussion and research findings make it clear that there are certain foods people are addicted to, and these foods—their very sight and smell — increases the metabolism in the brain. The food addiction does have a well defined scientific basis. Probably overeating, craving for food excessively (polyphagia), etc., may be related to these addictions. Modern science is yet to unravel these mysteries.

24

Health and Fitness

Many people find it very hard to start and stick to an exercise programme. The Allied Dunbar National Fitness Survey (1990) showed that seven out of 10 men, and eight out of 10 women do not do enough exercise. For many people, their views on sports and exercise were shaped during school PT lessons or through early involvement in sports. Sometimes as a result of these experiences, they are left with the impression that only strenuous sports and exercises are beneficial for health.

In fact there is a well-established body of knowledge that shows mild to moderate physical activity is the best way to a healthy lifestyle. So instead of asking how much exercise is good for him, a person asks how little can he get away with? For some people to think of doing a 30 minute brisk walk, or the practicalities of finding the time, is just too difficult. If this is the case, then he must consider accumulating this duration by shorter bouts of more frequent activity. Small steps to try:

1. Using the stairs rather than lift at work or in the shopping centre.

2. Parking the car/motorcycle farthest away from the entrance of the supermarket and not using the remote control to change TV channels.

3. Avoiding the too easy modern day gadgets whenever/
    wherever possible and trying to do work pending one's
    energy and thereby getting some physical activity.

Fitness has been defined in relation to a concept called
physical work capacity. This is related to how much work
the body can do. Fitness can be understood in relation to a
number of components such as endurance, flexibility, strength
and power. One needs to be fit to play many popular sports
such as football, hockey, squash, tennis.

Health is a broader concept that includes being free from
and resilient to disease, mental and spiritual well-being and
the quality of our social relationships. Normally being fit and
being healthy go hand in hand. But this is not always the
case. One can be very fit, through, for example, playing
football but be suffering from a major health problem like
alcoholism. Understanding the difference between health and
fitness is important because the level of exercise one needs to
do to be healthy is less than that which is needed to get and
keep him fit.

Training for Fitness

Many people need or want to be fit because of the job they do
(police officers), the sport they play (basketball) or because
they want to achieve a body shape that they aspire to, through
resistance training and other techniques.

If a person has to be fit them he normally needs to follow a
structured training programme. One of the key variables in
achieving a high level of fitness is the intensity of the exercise
programme. Of one wants to very fit then one needs to exercise
at a moderate or even higher intensity.

Common examples of fitness training includes circuits,
running and weight training. In achieving one's fitness goals
through these programmes most people will also become
healthier. However, if one doesn't need to be fit but just healthy
then one doesn't have to exercise as hard.

Being Active for Health

If a person wants to reduce his risk of suffering from coronary heart disease, obesity or other health problems then research indicates that he should be physically active. To achieve these health benefits it does not require the same intensity of exercise training that is required to become fit. One can simply build physical activity into one's daily living through, for example, brisk walking or cycling.

One can do this mild to moderate activity either as a form of 'active commuting' or in the comfort of a health club. Unfortunately, some people are put off becoming more active because they think they have to work out at a high intensity, compete with others or wear a designer tracksuit. None of these things are necessary. Even simple steps like taking the stairs instead of the lift can be a way of accumulating your weekly 'dose' of physical activity.

Staying Slender for Life

Eating what one likes is one of the most satisfying of life's pleasures for. Unfortunately excess weight often goes hand in hand with the joys of eating. It is very difficult for many people to take off and keep off that excess weight they acquire with time. A big reason is endless procession of quick fad diets. There are so many best selling fad diets and none of them work in the long run for the vast majority of people who try them. In fact, each new diet actually creates the demand for its successor. Millions may try a popular diet, even stick to it faithfully for a few weeks or months, and lose some weight, but sooner or later they tire of following someone else's formula, go off the diet, return to their old eating habits and regain the weight. When the next fad diet comes along, they are ready to try another magical ride on the weightless see saw say health experts.

Taking off weight should not be a temporary thing. It has to become a way of life—sensible eating and exercising habits that eventually become second nature to the person concerned.

Mild changes in eating habits can help one lose weight over a period of time. Consider the amount of weight one can lose in just one year by striving for these easily attainable diet goals

1. Eat just one pat less of butter or margarine daily and 1½ kilos disappear.

2. Cut out one slice of bread daily and off go more than 2½ kilos.

3. Omit just one bottle of beer once a week and at least 1 kilo goes away.

4. Skip 10 potato chips once a week and lose 100 gms.

5. Omit 2 slices of bacon once a week and 400 gms are cut.

6. Cut your sugar intake by 2 teaspoons a day and 1½ kilos are cut.

7. Omit just one piece of cake a week and 2½ kilos go away.

Depending on the person's lifestyle, metabolism and other factors if he eats just 100 calories more per day than what he needs to maintain the present weight, he/she would gain nearly half a kilo in five weeks → as much as 5 kilos in a year! Mild change of eating habits (like the ones given above) can easily reverse the above equation.

By a few strategic substitutions of lower calorie items in place of high calorie foods, a great difference can be made.

1. One must take boiled prawns (170 gms, 200 cal) instead of fried (170 gm, 380 gms) ones.

2. One must make broiled chicken (half chicken, 257 cal) rather than fried (half chicken, 464 calories).

3. One must substitute a parched or boiled egg for a fried egg for a 35 calorie saving.

4. One can substitute a slice of bacon for two strips of bacon for 31 saved calories.

5. One can take five sticks of raw carrots for five biscuits for saving of 85 calories.

One must consider portion sizes too. If a person loves a particular high calorie dish, it can be tough doing without it. An easier way is to have a smaller serving. One should prepare small pieces of meat, for example, and eat more vegetables and salad. Cooking methods also count. Whenever possible, foods should be broiled, basked, steamed or boiled—and fat to be trimmed away before cooking. The flavour of cooked foods can be enhanced without fat, by adding herbs or dry wine.

Exercise is also important for weight control, health and for staying trim and slim lifelong. It need not be extremely vigorous to be valuable. One can:

1. Jog in place.
2. Cycle at 20 km an hour.
3. Play handball.

In all these one will be expending 6-9 calories a minute. If these are done for 20 minutes a day, burning up as many as 180 calories one will lose 65,700 calories, the equivalent of more than 8 kilos in a year.

One can also take up lighter exercises.

1. Walking at a pace of 5 km an hour → 4 calories/minute are lost. If this is stepped up to 7 km/hr → 7 cal/minute are lost.

15 km an hour cycling
30 km/minute swimming $\Big]$ In both these activities 7 cal/minute expenditure is found.

But often a doubt expressed is: won't want a person eat more if he exercises more? Not necessarily, says new research. Although a thin person often will eat more after increased activity, the overweight person with stores of fat to draw upon may not experience an equivalent appetite increase after normal exercise.

First the general principles behind weight control must be understood. Then a specific plan must be implemented. One must never aim at more than half a kilo or a kilo loss a week. To lose that half a kilo one needs to decrease food intake and increase physical activity by 3,500 cal or 500 cal a day.

Some tips to eat less includes:

1. Drink more water.

2. Take more time and eat leisurely.

3. If there is no time to eat a leisurely meal, don't eat!

4. Eat more fibre rich, unrefined foods.

An average person, by the time he reaches his full maturity at 25 years will have started to put on weight that he doesn't need. And if he let himself gain even half a kilo a year, he will weigh 12½ kilos too much by the time he is 50. Keeping this calculation in mind one can just about understand that one never gets overweight with a rush. Overweight develops slowly over the years. One gets fat because of those extra calories that one sops up day by day beyond those one's body needs. 'To stay slender for life ' must be the aim and this can be achieved by the two magic words 'Exercise' and 'Diet'— both practised in a consistent and regular way.

Search for a Perfect Diet

People are always on the lookout for a perfect diet. If they are not talking about which eating plan to follow next they are worrying about what they have eaten. The obsession with weight has become so great that it often becomes the facial point of every action and reaction. And in many parts of the world it is also the age of permarexics. Permarexics encompass an entire generation of people who are constantly on a diet and their numbers are increasing by the hour. Unlike anorexics and bulimic, permarexics look at the world through a range of food restrictions. If they begin the day with the cornflakes diet, they might end it with the cabbage soup diet. They are constantly reading up information on fad diets and trying to find one that suits them. All day long, 365 days of the year, they are flitting from one food plan to the next.

There may be no shortcuts to becoming slim but there has not been no effort spared by dietitians and doctors alike to try and hit upon the perfect weight loss plan. 'No-starch diet', 'Wine and cheese diet' all are very popular with models and actors. Many popular celebrities stay way from strict diets and follow a relaxed but healthy diet. They say that basically it is important to be healthy and happy. Taking healthy food in the form of brown rice, whole wheat bread, oats, plenty of vegetables and fruits—these are their diet rules. 'Soya breaks down fats' is the latest belief and many youngsters include soya in their lunch and dinners. Soya milk has also become popular. Veggie diet Atkin's diets are followed by many. Some stick to them and others discard them after giving a brief try. 'To each his own' applies here.

'Fit for life diet' that says (1) Fruit should be eaten from the time you get up until noon as it helps to cleanse the system. Fruit should never be eaten with anything else. (2) For lunch and dinner one can either have a carbohydrate based meal which would be grains, beans and veggies or a protein meal which would be protein and veggies. Never combine carbohydrate and protein as they fight in the stomach and then become toxic. People gain weight not because of overeating and too little exercise but because they wrongly combine protein rich foods with starchy foods.

Many youngsters also prefer 'Zone diet' which is a bit liberal and combines protein, carbohydrates and fats.

Certain dietitians caution that fad diets can have ill effects on health in the long-term. They do more harm than good. Doctors say that cutting carbohydrates or only eating carbohydrates and various permutations over the years could weaken the system. Jaundice may attack such persons. Fitness consultants say that fad diets don't work because most of them are low in calories. Most diets allow the person to eat only one type of food. A person requires 1,800 cal and most diets offer far less than that. These diets don't have all the total food groups either. By following them a person may feel he has lost weight but actually he has lost only water. The body weight is a combination of lean body mass, fat, water weight. When he loses muscle the natural fat has not gone and when the diet is off, all of it comes back.

Fad diets are all the rage now. But nutritionists warn that they must be followed with caution. The ultimate and only workable diet they believe is about eating small and healthy meals and exercising regularly.

Here are some popular diets for interest's sake:

1. **Facial analysis diet**: Based on the principle that the secret to maintaining an ideal weight and health is written on a person's face. This personalised weight loss plan allows a facial analyst to pin point harmful and beneficial food by identifying a person's face type. Whether a person has lines on his forehead, red ears, thick tongue, large open pores—each requires a certain kind of diet.

2. **Sugar busters diet**: This diet requires a person to abstain from all refined sugar and processed grain products like wheatgrain and white rice. This claims to lower one's cholesterol, increase his energy and decrease health risks.

3. **The Mediterranean diet:** It involves high consumption of fruits, vegetables, bread and other cereals, potatoes, nuts and beans. Olive oil is an important monosaturated fat source. Dairy and red meat are low, eggs almost minimal and wine must be consumed in moderate amounts.

4. **The Stone Age diet**: The diet says the healthiest way to eat is to drop the modern day foods like diary food in favour of lean meat, fish, fruit, vegetables and nuts.

5. **GI diet**: The theory is that if one eats food with low Glycaemic Index (GI), one's blood sugar will stay balanced and one will have fewer cravings. Wholegrains and lentils are in, sugar, white bread, mashed potatoes and chocolates are out.

6. **Calorie restriction diet**: By reducing the calorie intake by 40 per cent, often having one meal a day, a person slows down the aging process to allow himself to live till 100 or more. The diet is big on flaxseed, rice bran, brewer's yeast, sprouts, with green tea and sugarfree gum for snacks.

7. **Weight watcher's diet:** The goal here is to help people make healthy eating decisions and encourage them to enjoy more physical activity. Each food is assigned points and the person concerned is allotted a certain number of points each day. By increasing activity and cutting back on calories, a dieter can keep his or her weight from increasing even more.

8. **Zone diet**: According to this diet, the ideal ratio of carbohydrates, proteins and fats is 40:30:30 respectively. There are two methods one can use to control the portion size of carbohydrates and proteins. One has to eat one's first meal or snack within an hour of waking and the last meal an hour before going to sleep at night.

The da Vinci Diet

Created by Stephen Lanzalotta, a baker who lost customers after the Atkin's diet hit the popularity chart, it is based on the mathematical value of 'phi' popularised by Dan Brown's worldwide bestseller **The da Vinci Code**. Lanzalotta argues that the links of human civilisation and grain have been around too long to be dismissed and that bread is a building block to stable moods, cleaner thoughts and the washboard abs of a renaissance statue. The diet focuses on MEDITERRANEAN food with the important add-on of bread and, unlike the Atkin's diet does not choose to change the biochemistry of the body.

25

Obesity in Children

Rising affluence among middle class families in producing a generation of obese children. Parents need to know that the price of their children's corpulence is heavy. Overweight kids are highly prone to a host of diseases and conditions. Screening programmes conducted by certain hospitals found that obese students who weigh about twice their ideal weight were at significantly higher risk for diabetes, high cholesterol, and high blood pressure. Though statistics are coming from different parts of the world, an accurate statistics from Singapore says that about 12 per cent of school children in Singapore are overweight! An interesting report from Philippines says that the number of obese Filipino kids referred to pediatric endocrine clinics is increasing. A decade ago only a few referrals would come to the specialists and now certain doctors attend to about one to four patients a month! Undernutrition was always a problem of great intensity in the Philippines but now overnutrition is on the rise too!

Bane of Modern Living

Our modern lifestyle has become a bane to children's health. Rather than play sports outdoors a lot of kids spend most of the day at home watching DVD movies or beating the highest score in the newest playstation game. With both parents working full time, kids often have free rein over what they eat. To make up for the little time they spend with their kids on weekdays, parents pander to their children's liking for junk food during weekend outings. Poor eating habit is a major cause of obesity among children. A sedentary lifestyle compounds the problem. Kids are eating more high calorie fast foods, spending more time in the front of the computer monitor and TV screen and less time on physical activities. This applies to kids all around the world.

A belief popular among many parents is that plump kids with their chubby cheeks and cuddly looks are more adorable. They also believe that "healthy" children will eventually shed the excess pounds as they mature. The truth is, obese childern do not readily lose weight as they grow older. Research shows that overweight adolescents have a 70 per cent chance of becoming overweight or obese adults.

Obesity has a negative impact on a child's psychological development. Children who are overweight face social pressures in school. They tend to fare poorly in sports and may feel they are not as physically attractive as their peers. "Overweight kids need helps", say doctors. In the past corpulence was regarded as a sign of prosperity and this belief still holds true in certain cultures. Today thin is beautiful and this a message largely media driven and perpetuated by ultraslim models and actress on magazine covers and TV. Overweight kids get teased and bullied physically and verbally which can result in a traumatic childhood. They may even develop obstructive sleep apnea, which affects their quality of sleep. As a result they suffer from poor concentration at school, which further erodes their self-image. People with sleep apnea literally stop breathing repeatedly during their sleep, often for a minute or longer and as many as hundreds of times during a single night.

Some kids may look fat but are actually healthy. The best way to find out if your child's weight is within the normal range is by measuring his body mass index or BMI. BMI is a measure of body fat based on height and weight—i.e., your child's weight in kilograms divided by the square of his height in metres.

Health professionals often use a BMI growth chart to assess whether a child or adolescent is overweight. For children the percentage ideal body weight for height (% IBW) or BMI is used. A person needs to check the weight and height of his child and plot it on the percentage IBW or BMI chart in his child's health book or at his doctor's clinic. A percentage IBW of more than 140 or BMI of more than 85th percentile for age and sex (qualifies as) obesity. He must talk to a pediatrician to find out more about his child's BMI and percentage IBW.

What Parents can do

1. Keep a close watch on your children's diet. Provide them with foods recommended in the food pyramid. Avoid empty calories—sweets, sodas, fried foods, foods with thick gravy, etc. Encourage them to opt for steamed, boiled or grilled foods instead.

2. Give your children lots of fresh fruits, vegetables, and wholegrains. For a treat give them fruit instead of candy. Serve water instead of sodas.

3. Make exercise a family affair. Go cycling or swimming take walks in the park. Physical activity burns calories and improves overall health. If your child sees you enjoying healthy foods and physical activity, he is more likely to do the same now and for the rest of his life.

4. Focus on your child's health and positive qualities, not your child's weight. Try not to make him feel different. Let him know he is loved and appreciated whatever his weight. Overweight children are probably more aware than anyone else that they have a weight problem. They need support, acceptance and encouragement. Parents should give their overweight kids lots of love. Emphasise that values are more important, not looks.

5. Gradually change your family's physical activity and eating habits. Slowly introduce good food choices.

Instead of removing all unhealthy foods, try reducing the portions first. If your kids feel deprived, they may crave for more.

6. Lead by example. Read up about nutrition. Teach your kids to read food labels.

7. Establish regular eating times. Eat only at the dining table and not in front of the TV. Limit snacks.

8. Reduce the amount of time you and your family spend in sedentary activities such as watching TV or playing video games.

9. Help your overweight children maintain their current weight growing normally in height.

10. If the child is morbidly obese, seek your doctors' advice. The child will require proper supervision for weight loss as well as diagnosis and management of associated diseases.

Parents and Schools Team up

In the 90's the Trim and Fit programme was started in Singapore schools to reduce obesity and improve physical fitness among pupils. Parents were asked to encourage their kids to participate in their school's 'nutrition and exercise programme'. Parents were cautioned about working late during week days, and during weekends giving children a treat by taking them to a fast food restaurant encourages obesity. Many overweight children shed their extra kilos after joining their school exercise programmes. Eating becomes more disciplined as the children learn the consequences of overweight in the nutrition programmes.

Why can't such programmes be included in schools of other countries also? India can definitely do with such programmes in its schools. Are the school principals listening?

26

Foods That Fight Fat

The idea that some foods can magically melt kilos away has been around for a long time. Of course, while exercise and a variety of wholesome foods are the secret to long-term weight control, there are foods that help us burn calories and quash hunger pangs. The following section discusses 10 such food items that helps stop overeating and stay healthy.

1. **Spinach**: Foods such as raw spinach contain bulk; so the space they fill in our stomach partly because of their high water content leaves less room for pastries and ice-cream. They are also crammed with iron, foliate, calcium and vitamins A, B, C, E. Certain research studies point out that women eating plenty of foliate rich foods significantly reduce the risk of giving birth to a child with cleft lip or palate.

2. **Grapefruit**: They are powerful 'fat fighters' due to their fibre content and without added sugar, a grapefruit has fewer calories than an orange of the same weight. In addition, the phyto chemicals and soluble fibre in citrus fruits lower cholesterol.

3. **Apples**: Eating several apples a day is a great idea. Hard fruits like apples take time to chew and fill one up. (One small glass of juice, however, contains the calories of about

two apples). Recent studies say that those who ate foods high in flavinoids found in fruit, vegetables and especially apples and oranges were 20 per cent less likely to suffer a stroke.

4. **Celery:** A person burns more calories chewing and digesting celery than it actually contain. Celery has vitamins E and C. It is a diet food but it should be on everyone's plate. Vegetables high in phyto chemicals (celery, broccoli) can help prevent cancer.

5. **Black Beans**: Protein-packed legumes such as black beans, chickpeas and lentils are not just low in fat and rich in soluble fibre, they digest slowly and keep blood sugar levels steady. One doesn't feel like refuelling for a while. Regularly eating black or navy beans may lower one's risk of colon cancer.

6. **Chillies:** Capsaicin, the compound that is found in chilies, does boost our metabolism slightly, increasing the energy our body burns during digestion. But a person should not make his food so hot that he will want to wash it down with a basketful of bread. Eating capsaicin may curb our appetite for three hours.

7. **Low fat milk:** Calcium rich foods do seem to boost metabolism. Researchers have found that women and girls who consume dairy products regularly have lower weight and less body fat than those who don't. Women consuming plenty of calcium-rich dairy foods slashed their overran cancer risk by 54 per cent, says a preliminary American study done in 2002.

8. **Mackarel:** Omega 3 fatty fish like mackerel, hilsa and sardines are all considered good for health. The protein mixed with fat in these fishes signals the brain, "That's enough" and curbs hunger. The mistake many dieters make is to cut out fat completely. Fat is what makes one

feel full. Overweight and hypertensive subjects who ate fish daily saw their blood fats drop and 'good' cholesterol rise as revealed by an Australian study programme.

9. **Cottage Cheese:** Cottage cheese (paneer) has much less fat than cheddar cheese. Cottage cheese is also a very good source of protein. The white curds are also stuffed with calcium, Vitamin B$_{12}$, zinc and foliate. Riboflavin found in paneer guards against anaemia and cancer, according to an American hospital study.

10. **Strawberries:** While all fruits contain vitamins, some are bigger nutritional winners than others. Strawberries, peaches, plums and grapes come with cancer fighting carotenoids and appetite suppressing fibre. But watermelon, pineapple, muskmelon and papaya fly through our system and cause our blood sugar to spike. One must aim for five or 10 servings of fruits and vegetables a day, choosing more of the winners. Research studies state that eating at least three servings of fruit and vegetables a day shrank the odds of dying from heart disease by 24 per cent.

Two topics here need to be discussed

(1) The weight packers (2) Protein foods.

1. Weight packers

Studies suggest that the combination of fructose and dextrose can interfere with our brain's ability to recognise we are full. 'Reduce the sugar intake in general', recommend diet experts. Extra sugar in our body in stored as fat. So we must choose whole fruit over dried, and fruit canned in its own juice instead of syrup. Hydrogenated fats (vanaspati) are another no-no. Unlike the non-unsaturated fats in some cooking oils or the polyunsaturated fats in nuts and seeds—the good fats—hydrogenated fats are found in processed foods such as pastries, french fries and biscuits. When hydrogen gas is added to otherwise healthy unsaturated liquid fat, it turns into a solid, partly saturated 'trans fat' that can send our bad cholesterol levels, heart disease risk, and weight sky rocketing. We must avoid these fats whenever possible. One can start by skipping fried foods. The medical experts, dietitians and nutritionists— all the three recommend this.

2. Protein Foods

Will protein foods curb our cravings? This is a common question asked by everyone. Let us see the views of dietitians. Proteins have a role in making us feel full, say diet experts. Proteins take longer to digest than carbohydrates. But many people make the mistake of not balancing their protein intake throughout the day. They wait till until the dinner time at which points they fill up on meat or other protein-rich foods. At lunch time they will eat a vegetable sandwich or salad but will get hungry again by mid-afternoon. This is not correct. The nutritionists suggest making protein work for a person throughout the day by adding some chicken, fish (or low fat dairy products) to that lunch-time veggie salad or sandwich. Or add some extra ham to that ham sandwich. These suggestions must be followed for balancing our protein intake throughout the day. Further, the experts say that if we eat toast with jam for breakfast, we must add natural peanut butter to it to keep us going longer. Such easy-to-follow tips can go a long way in making our diet a balanced and nutritious one.

Obesity and Teenage (Indian Scene)

Sleek, well toned bodies, fab abs, the perfect figure...they are everywhere. We see them in ads, on the big screen, on bill boards, and in magazines. So why talk about obesity? Ask teenagers. The answer is the real picture is very different. If diets are in, so are fast food joints and aerated drinks. And the fight against flab is a REAL struggle, especially for today's youth.

The rise in obesity among teenagers is significant, say medical experts. The number of obese teenagers in the four metros of India is rising nearly one in five or six teenagers has an obesity problem. Why metros? They are the ones directly affected by the influx of Western culture. In even rural populations where fast food joints have opened up, obesity is on the rise. For example, in the north-east, there are little towns where fast food joints have opened. These populations mirror the obesity of the towns.

So should we cut pizzas, colas, burgers, and potato chips totally out of our diet? Your lifestyle is also to blame, specially if you have a sedentary lifestyle or do not exert yourself physically.

Why should one worry about obesity? Doctors say simply because India suffers under the double burden of disease-malnutrition on one hand and obesity on the other. Regarding the Indian population as a whole, about 5 to 7 per cent of the high and middle income group of the Indian population is obese. A small percentage may be, but what is of the concern is that they also make the cream of society. They make up the most productive workforce consisting of academicians, planners and politicians. Hence the need to address the issue before it blows up into an unmanageable crisis.

Obesity is the major risk factors for non-communicable diseases. Both parents and doctors are worried about the ill health packages that come along with obesity. Obese teenagers become obese adults. And they are at greater risk for diseases like heart disease, stroke, lung failure, kidney failure, hypertension, type II diabetes. Previously, a large number of people in the age group of 30 to 40 got heart attacks. That has now advanced to youngsters of 25 or 26!

For the morbidly obese sometimes surgery is the only option. Bariatric surgery restricts the stomach capacity so that the person experiences early satiety, says a surgeon in Chennai who has performed 16 such surgeries in the last three to four years! The surgery is ideal when done on patients between 20 and 54, since it can reverse a lot of processes in the body. Many such operated cases have got cured of their diabetes. But these surgeries have risks and definitely not a cosmetic surgery.

Being 'huge' can also lead to depression in teenagers. Certain consultant doctors for children and adolescents say that the term obese is no longer politically correct. They categorise it as 'tendency to be overweight' and 'overweight'. Most of these consultants feel that one cannot ask an adolescent to eat less. What should be done is reduce inactivity and the sedentary pattern of life. School-based health services is the need of the hour. Hospitals should have a special way of dealing with obese adolescents.

Modern medicine is coming up with ways to help the overweight. But self-help is the best help. By being just a little cautious one can help oneself a lot.

Calorie Tips for Teenagers

1. When you eat food look at it as simple (eg. sugar, cake) and complex (vegetabes, fruits chappatis) calories. Develop a taste for complex calories.

2. Avoid rice, oil, and sugar.

3. Exercise regularly.

4. Avoid aerated drinks; they are just a empty calories.

5. It is fine to eat burgers or pizzas once in a while. Have them everyday and you are asking for trouble.

6. Opt for high protein, low carbohydrate and zero fat diet.

'Self check' for Obesity

No teenager should let the mirror tell him whether he is obese. Instead, he must rely on simple maths. The same old trustsworthy BMI.

$$BMI= \frac{wt \text{ in kg}}{\text{Square of height in m.}}$$

If BMI is above 25 → the person is obese.

If BMI is above 30 → significantly obese.

If BMI is above 40 → morbidly obese.

27

Pregnancy and Weight Gain

It is common to see the mother (or the husband in the present day context) fussing over the diet of the pregnant woman. While the 'mothers to-be' enjoy basking in the attention showered upon them, it is essential that they take care of their nutrition, for the health of the child is very much dependent on the mother's diet.

Pregnancy and weight gain

Normal weight gain during pregnancy is 10 to 12 kg.

Pregnancy is a time when appetite is altered and nutritional needs change. What the expectant mother eats or drinks can affect her baby's health. Though underweight (10% less than ideal weight) is not desirable, obesity in pregnancy increases the risk of mother developing hypertension and diabetes during pregnancy.

122

Normal weight gain during pregnancy is usually around 10 to 12 kgs but obese patients should not put on more than 7.7 to 8 kgs overall during pregnancy. Nutritional requirements vary from individual to individual and each stage of pregnancy has special requirements. A pregnant woman's requirement is about 2500 cal/day and her diet should include 100 gms of protein, 100 gms of fat and three glasses of milk besides plenty of green leafy vegetables and fruits. For patients who can't tolerate milk, high calcium foods such as yoghurt and cheese are substituted.

Meat is a rich source of iron and protein. And for vegetarians nuts and legumes are adequate. It is a common practice to prescribe iron, calcium, folic acid, vitamin D and other trace elements like zinc. One should be cautioned against overdose of nutrients, as it could prove harmful during pregnancy. However, food articles like pickles should not be taken. Nausea and vomiting during pregnancy have a serious impact on the physical and emotional aspects of the woman's life.

Morning sickness is not always experienced in the morning. Commonly women develop an aversion for fried food, coffee and some even experience a craving for sweet food and sometimes craving for non-food items like coal, soap, etc., but this must be discouraged.

If a patient has the inability to retain any solid or liquid food with electrolyte imbalance the condition is called 'Hypermesis gravidarum'. It requires prompt attention. Constipation is common during pregnancy. So pregnant women should be advised to add more roughage like bran and cereals.

General advice is to eat healthy food but drink lots of water. Also heart burn is common during pregnancy, so usual meal pattern of three square meals is unsuitable. It is good to have five or even six small meals throughout the day.

Tips for being Mobile and Independent

- Raise the level of chair/ toilet seats/ beds as it as difficult to get up from low chairs.

- Water and wax therapy which serves to grease joints.

- Using a stick fixed with a hook to pick up objects instead of bending.

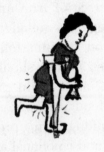

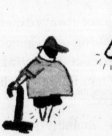
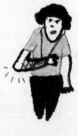

"LOSE WEIGHT"

OR

ARTHRITIS MAY

JUST CRIPPLE YOU

28

Obesity and Arthritis

The Ultimatum

'Lose weight or arthritis may just cripple you' warn medical experts. This ultimatum has lot of substantial evidence. If a woman 'on the heavier side' presents herself, her chances of arthritis stand at 7 out of 10! Also a consensus of doctors puts the incidence of women being more prone than men at 7 out of 10.

And being a progressively degenerative disorder, arthritis is not fatal but crippling for life. The Arthritis Foundation of India established in 1995 offers a network for those afflicted with arthritis, in the form of tips on manoeuvering in everyday situation.

There are two types of arthritis and people often get confused between the two. Rheumatoid arthritis which, according to doctors, is affecting younger women of late, is stated as 'auto immune disease' wherein the body's own antibodies starts fighting against connecting tissues, especially joints. It is so incapacitating that it just cripples a person overnight and he doesn't know what to do with himself. For young women of child-bearing age, it becomes a crisis.

Physiotherapists feel there are ways of overcoming the pain and subsequent deformities, though to a small extent. Certain orthetic devices have been designed to make the affected person carry out his work independently. There are also some muscle strengthening ways to mobilise joint manually and through electric adjuncts. The weather of certain places (*e.g.*, Bangalore, in India) makes the people arthritic.

Indian women tend to be heavier than men and hence develop slight bow legs during their middle age. Rheumatoid arthritis spreads to the whole body, Osteoarthritis is due to wear and tear. Actually 10 per cent to 15 per cent people worldwide have some form of arthritis. It is insidious and comes with no warning.

One message that is loud and clear is one must lose weight, otherwise arthritis is bound to cripple him.

The Concept of Muscle Toning

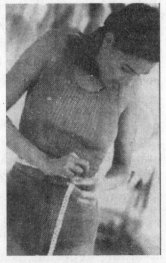

'Toning' is a word created by the fitness industry to attract women to lifting weights. Their idea is to acquire a well toned body, not a big bulky body. How does a person get toned? By lifting weights seriously; not doing a few easy sets of 10 to 20 reps with pink plastic dumbbells. Toning is about gaining lean muscle mass. But for some reason women are afraid of that and think they are going to look like the incredible hulk. The word was made up just for women who have these fears. Often, women who want to get 'toned' will overwhelm their bodies with a variant of exercise reps, sets and no consistency in their workouts.

There are no two ways about it. In order to achieve the look of muscle tone or toned body a person needs to engage in strength training as well as shed the layer of fat covering his muscles. Just because he is not looking to get bulky or add muscle mass doesn't mean that he should shy away from strength training. He needs to put in some effort and his muscles need to be stressed in order for them to change and grow. The myth of toning is often tangled in the myth of spot training. Someone might say that he wants to tone the back of his arms and so he is going to do some triceps exercises. He can do it of course. He can work his triceps but that isn't going to get rid of the fat around his triceps. Which is what keeps him from seeing that muscle. If he reduces his calories, lifts weights and does some cardio he can lose body fat. Can he then lose it over his triceps? Sure, he can! But only his body will decide when (or if) the fat over that particular area will go.

Developing those Lone Handles

Developing a lean, flat stomach takes time and patience especially when it comes to those last few pounds in those hard to lose places. The 'lower abs' and 'lone handles' can be two of the most stubborn and exercise resistant areas from which to lose fat. In fact it can sometimes seem so hard to reduce those spots that many people became frustrated and resort to dangerous diet, drugs or liposuction.

There is only one way to lose fat in the 'stubborn areas' and that is with the correct combination of proper diet, cardiovascular exercise, abdominal training and weight training. The first thing one needs to realise is that it is impossible to spot reduce fat from one specific part of the body. Achieving a toned tummy and being able to actually see that muscle tone is to get rid of the layer of body fat covering one's abs.

It doesn't matter how many crunches one does or what a new machine one uses from the advertisements that one sees every day. If a person doesn't reduce his body fat, he will never see those strong toned abs.

Contrary to popular belief the best way to burn the layer of flab from one's mid-section is not to do more abdominal exercise but to do more right kind of cardiovascular exercises. Even if one is doing cardio every day without a good diet he still won't see results. Fat loss in a 50 per cent exercise and 50 per cent nutrition combination. Regardless of how much a person works out, if the number of calories he takes in is greater than the amount he burns, he will still put on weight.

29

Cut Those Carbohydrates

The average birth weight of a baby varies across the globe from 2,400 gm to 4,000 gm. Babies

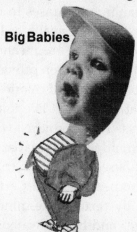

Big Babies

Babies above 400 gm are considered high birth weight called Macrosomia

above 4,000 gm are considered as high birth weight. And the term used is <u>Macrosomia.</u> It is associated with maternal and foetal trauma at delivery and a doubling of the parental mortality rate. Heavy babies can result from foetal diseases like 'Anasarca' (whole body edoema) in infants, with erythroblastosis foetalis (rh incompatible baby). Excess growth antenatally follow conditions such as cerebral gigantism, transposition of great vessels, Beckwith Wiedemann syndrome.

Classically maternal diabetes is linked to large babies but studies show that abnormal glucose tolerance is present in only a minority of mothers of large babies. Big women tend to have big babies. Macrosomia is also common in women who have had a large infant before, especially if they are over 35 years

Diagnosis before birth depends on suspicion. Ultra -scanning for weight prediction is less accurate at extremes of body size but it helps. Most foetal deaths and damages cannot be prevented but injuries associated with delivery of macrosomic infants can be prevented. Macrosomia is associated with neonatal trauma. Meconium aspiration, asphyxia and brachial plexus injuries occur. Preventing high birth weight by dietary restriction in pregnancy caesarean section seems to be the indication due to the potential dangers of vaginal delivery. Elective (well-planned) surgery is the safest procedure and one need not wait up to the emergency stage.

Healthy Proverbs

It is time to add new and more meaningful phrases to our store of proverbs that teach us how to lead a healthier life. Most of the health programmes and schemes are meant to create a healthy living. People often remember proverbs although they may not remember tables of data of calories or metabolic rates. Proverbs such as 'eat to live, not live to eat' were created by our great grandparents. A few hundred years down the road, we will be the great grandparents. Maybe we have to create new health proverbs based on clinical trials, rather than observations that haven't been verified Certain health proverbs have been created by certain like-minded individuals to spread health messages and bring awareness. They reflect today's public health principles providing advice on such things as:

1. Quit smoking.

2. Maintain a balanced diet.

3. Being physically active.

   Their modern proverbs include:

1. The more you smoke, the more you croak (to quit smoking).

2. A tri colour meal is a good deal (nutrition, encouraging you to eat red, yellow and green fruits and vegetables).

3. Seven days without exercise makes one weak (to stress physical activity importance).

See how beautifully the word 'weak' has been used to substitute the four days week. This proverb condemns all the couch potatoes (sedentary T.V watchers) and 'mouse' potatoes (a person lazily glued to his computer for a long time).

A proverb is usually a homely illustration of a great truth and is not meant to be a dry scientific statement.

'Porridge gives you a edge' (stresses advantage of a porridge). Porridge might prove to be a very healthy breakfast dish, say researchers. It also reduces risk of a heart attack. Being high in fibre, low in sugar, salt and fat it should be an ideal choice for dieters. It also releases carbohydrates slowly into the body; it is being advocated as an essential part of the new GI (glycaemic index) diet. This makes one feel full and prevents one from reaching for the chocolate, biscuits before lunch time. As it is made with milk, it is also a great way to boost calcium intake.

Cut Those Carbohydrates

Moving to low carbohydrate diet doesn't mean just giving up meat for pasta or egg for morning bread. The following section lists 12 useful tips to make the changeover or shift from the usual high carbohydrate meal to a low carb diet, a smooth one.

1. Count the carbohydrates. When a person eats carbohydrate he must go in for complex ones like wholegrain breads and pasta, pulses and non-starchy vegetables and fruits.

2. Go for foods that lower glucose response. Fruits and vegetables that have the lowest glycemic index are apples, apricots, broccoli and asparagus.

3. Read food labels. Food labels have to show the grams of carbohydrates each serving contains. One must read the food labels carefully and keep track of the carbohydrates in the various foods consumed.

4. Avoid soft drinks. Soda, sweetened juices, aerated drinks are storehouses of low quality carbohydrates. One must stick to iced tea (no sugar) or water when one feels thirsty.

5. Stock up on low carb food. One must fill one's fridge and kitchen with non-starchy foods, fruits, vegetables, fish, dairy products so that snack time is also easier.

6. Plan ahead. If one has to eat out, one must go to a restaurant that offers more than breads or pasta, a seafood joint, for example.

7. Nutty nuts. Peanuts and other nuts are full of monosaturated fats and help contribute to weight loss and hearty health.

8. Change cooking oils. One must choose monosaturated oils like peanut oil, olive oil, canola oil for cooking and salad dressing. They are healthier for the heart.

9. Keep an eye on the sauces. Relishes, sauces and ketchup are chockfull of carbs, up to 4 gms of carbohydrates per tablespoon. Barbecue sauces have up to 8 gms!

10. Stick to lean meats. Just because one is switching to a low carb diet one need not gorge on fatty meats. These have high levels of saturated fats (bad for the heart). One must opt for lean beef, pork, and poultry. One must remove the skin and any fat one can see.

11. Fishing around, one must try seafood instead. It is rich in protein, and omega 3 fatty acids which are polyunsaturated fatty acids that protect against heart attack and are important for brain and nerve cells. Higher fat, cold water fish like mackerel, tuna, salmon, sardines, and lake trout are full of omega 3 fatty acids.

12. Move. No matter what diet one is on, one must exercise. It increases metabolism and flexibility, burns calories and strengthens muscles, improves circulation, and one's mood. There are many more such benefits. The aim must be 30 minutes moderate exercise a day. Combined with a healthy, low carb diet, one can lose weight and stay healthy.

Nutritional Myths

We grow up thinking something is true and never question until someone comes along and tells us our thinking was wrong. We must learn the new things even if they fly in the face of what mom taught us.

1. Cottage cheese is not a good source of calcium. Hard cheeses usually have two to four times as much calcium as cottage cheese, and milk and yoghurt are still the best (300 to 400 mg per cup). Cottage cheese is still a good source of protein and is much lower in fat than other cheeses. This makes it a good food to include in our diet but not as a major source of calcium.

2. Vine ripened tomatoes are not necessarily more nutritious tomatoes. They may taste better than the kind that are shipped green, then gassed with a plant hormone called ethylene to complete the maturing process. But the amounts of vitamin C and Beta carotene are nearly the same.

3. Eating lots of sugar does not cause diabetes. But being overweight does tend to increases the risk of having diabetes. If one is overweight primarily because of one's sugar intake than the two may be related.

4. Drinking carbonated liquids when one is nauseated will not make him feel better. In fact, all fluids, especially the bubbly ones, are hard to keep down when somebody's stomach is upset. The better remedy is a cracker or other dry food.

5. Fresh squeezed juices are good for us. But they are not better than whole fruits and vegetables. They cannot cure arthritis, migraine or other chronic maladies. Salesmen who sell expensive juicers would have one believe that juices are medicines. They are not. Ounce for ounce, the juice of an orange has as much vitamin C as an orange but would lose some other nutrients that remain in the solids. In the case of carrot juice one carrot has less beta-carotene than a cup of carrot juice because it takes more than one to make a cup of juice. But would lose the fibre unless the carrot is pureed.

6. Vitamins do not provide quick energy. Vitamins do not have any calories and thus provide no energy at all. The only way to get energy is by eating carbohydrates, fats and proteins. Many vitamins are co-enzymes, which means that they work with other nutrients to release energy. But the body can only use a certain quantity of vitamins and if one takes more than one's body can absorb the excess will be excreted or stored in fat.

Don't Fall for the Diet Hype

Along with the nutritional myths one needs some clarification on the advertisements that promise one will lose pounds quickly and effortlessly. We are seeing so many "get slim quick" promotions everywhere that we seem to get brain-washed. Though many of these are genuine and credible; some are false and misleading. Many false diet claims are increasing in statistics.

Health experts recommend that one should ignore the hype, and make lifestyle changes instead. A person is setting himself up for failure if he believes the ads that tell him that it is easy to lose weight. It isn't. Nor is it fast. In fact, rapid weight loss is the sign of a poorly designed diet. When one is losing weight rapidly one is losing muscle and protein.

There is an exception when one first goes on a diet. One can lose five or six pounds, that is primarily water. That rapid weight loss diminishes after the first week. If one is eating a balanced diet of fruits, vegetables, wholegrains, lean meat and poultry, one's weight loss should taper to a pound or two a week. At that rate it will take about six months to lose 30 pounds, which isn't exciting enough to advertise but could mean a permanent and healthier weight loss.

Experts recommend the following criteria to determine whether to use a diet product or programme:

1. One should ask about the success rate of the plan; if the information is not available, one should not go on that diet.

2. One must avoid a diet regimen that promises one will never go hungry and one will always be full. That is not a valid diet promise.

3. One should be sceptical about 'before' and 'after' pictures.

4. One should not follow a diet that prohibits certain food groups. That is a shortsighted way to eat. One may gorge on those forbidden foods later.

30

Obesity Unbound

Obesity Galore

- Obesity is not a 'restricted to this area' problem.
- It is a worldwide problem.
- It is present everywhere in the world.
- It has no geographical favourites.
- Lifestyle changes everywhere have led to globalisation of obesity.

Obesity in a Nutshell

- Obesity is excessive body fat, but this is difficult to measure directly. For this reason body mass index (BMI), which is a measure of weight, corrected for differences in height, is most commonly used to define obesity. BMI is computed as weight (in kg) divided by height squared (in metres). The WHO has defined BMI of 30 or greater as obesity.

- Overweight is defined as a BMI of 25 to 29.9. Although the health risks for being overweight, including diabetes, heart disease, and some cancers, are less than those for obesity, they are still substantial.

Visitors to the United States are often struck by the signs of obesity seen everywhere. In Europe, indeed, the old stereotype of the "ugly American" tourist is being replaced by the caricature of the "Fat American". Certain statistics show that the percentage of American adults who are obese increased from 12 per cent in 1991 to 18 per cent in 1998. Another large fraction of American population is also above a healthy weight but below the formal definition of obesity. Half of all Americans indeed are either overweight or are obese by World Health Organisation (WHO) standards. Obesity rates in children are also raising fast.

The obesity epidemic is global, and includes many East European and developing countries, for example, the rates for being overweight and obese in Mexico, Kuwait and South Africa are similar to or exceed those in America. In Russia, surveys show that 30 to 35 per cent of women and 10 to 15 per cent of men are obese. In Germany, obesity rates are 20 to 30 per cent for women and 15 to 20 per cent for men.

No longer is obesity a luxury of the rich; instead it is an affliction of the poor. In affluent countries, indeed, obesity is now two or three times more likely in people with the lowest educational attainment.

The health consequences and the costs incurred in treating the complications arising from obesity and excess weight are enormous. In America, excess body fat account for about 90 per cent of adult onset of diabetes, about one-third of heart attacks, contributes to several major cancers, arthritis, cataracts and reduced quality of life in general. Disconcertingly, the form of diabetes previously only seen in adults is now commonly seen in adolescents.

Although genetic factors influence the likelihood of obesity, they cannot explain such massive increases in so short a period of time. Fundamentally, weight gain occurs when physical activity decreases or total calorie intake increases. Obesity as an epidemic should come as no surprise because many aspects of contemporary life promote it.

Convenient transport and sedentary occupations dramatically reduced physical activity throughout the world. Eighty per cent of the world's population now has access to sufficient food, says a September 2001 statistics. A great accomplishment, but consuming even a small amount of food above what is necessary will lead to obesity within a few years. With opportunities to eat ever present—ast food shops, readymade dinner — the human weakness to indulge is fully exploited.

What should be done? We should first recognise that obesity does not come from eating fat. People eat less fat now and are more obese than ever. Indeed, medical trials show that fat and carbohydrates have similar effects on body fat. So those faddish no fat, high carbohydrate diets are doomed to fail. The urban poor in developing countries show that high rates of obesity occur when limited physical activity is combined with simple starchy diets.

How can obesity be controlled? Although many dream of a pill to cure the problem, a safe and effective drug does not exist. So instead of looking for a magic wand we should recognise that obesity is a function of social change: urbanisation, sedentary lives, and the consumption of mass-produced high calorie foods.

In principle, if every individual exercised regularly and was careful about calorie intake obesity would be uncommon. But because low levels of physical activity and over-consumption are deeply imbedded in our lifestyles, individuals acting in isolation face many obstacles. An effective strategy to fight the obesity epidemic will require both individual and Institutional initiatives.

1. Nutritionists must provide improved dietary advice and make it accessible to all.

2. Health care providers can do more to counsel patients about the importance of minimising weight gain as adults.

3. Schools and businesses can require daily physical activity, serve healthy meals and integrate health education into their routines.

4. Parents can limit television watching, computer-related lazy activities like browsing, etc. Parents can also avoid buying soft drinks. They should express love without high calorie sweets and must be good role models in their diets.

5. Governments can provide facilities for safe walking, bicycle transportation and recreation.

Although we willingly spend massive amounts of money to treat the diseases and health complications that arise when so many people are so overweight we are reluctant to invest even modestly in strategies that can prevent the underlying problem. This must change if the obesity epidemic is to be contained.

Preventive strategies are particularly important in poor countries. During the next 30 years, United Nations demographers predict that two billion people will be added to the world's population. The large majority will be in poor urban areas of developing countries, places where some of the largest increases in obesity are now being recorded and where provision of expensive medical care is difficult. Sadly these cities are typically expanding without including safe facilities for recreation. Such facilities are not expensive to include when streets are being created but are costly to build retrospectively. They should be required components of all urban planning.

Can prevention work? Many individuals, having learned to exercise and avoid excessive calorie intake, are controlling their weight. The shift of the obesity burden from the rich to the poor in many Western countries demonstrate that knowledge and the ability to act upon it are important. We also have examples of countries—Holland and some Scandinavian countries—where exercise is encouraged by the inclusion of bicycles and pedestrians in urban design. The obesity epidemic can be controlled, but everyone's effort is needed.

Overcoming Overweight

That *Lancet Medical Journal* calls obesity a time bomb that is ticking away. There have been so many drugs, so many techniques to cure obesity but all these countless wonder drugs and magic techniques vanished as fast as they appeared. Scientists are trying to control overweight and obesity by newer tactics. A drug called 'Orlistat' is considered a milestone in the treatment of obesity. It works not by the usual mechanism of suppressing the opposite but by blocking an enzyme that helps digestion and absorption of fat. The enzyme is known as lipase, which is secreted by the pancreas as part of the pancreatic juice. This juice is in fact a major digestant as it takes care of digesting and absorbing the three major nutrients needed by the body, namely, carbohydrates, fats and, proteins.

It will be surprising to know that, contrary to the drastic weight reduction promised by countless health care touts, the scientific community is prepared to accept only 10 per cent reduction in body weight in obese patients as proof of efficacy, since the body resorts to what are known as 'counter regulatory mechanisms' that do not allow the body weight to fall below this level easily. If a drug produces a 10 per cent weight loss as compared to the baseline and if it produces more weight loss than a dummy medicine known as placebo in medical jargon, then it can be given registration as an antiobesity agent, state the guidelines of official European Medicines Evaluation Agency.

When we are talking of obesity, we are not simply talking of one single number that appears on a person's weighing scale or the card that pops out of the weighing machine in railway stations. There is more to the problem of obesity than mere kilograms and pounds. The scientific index BMI (body mass index) is used by nutritional scientists in this connection. It is obtained by dividing bodyweight in kilos by the square of height in metres. The BMI is supposed to be between 18.5 and 25 kg per sqm for normal persons. Values between 25 and 30 are seen in overweight persons and more than 30 in frank obesity.

Going by BMI, the whole world seems to be getting obese. The number of persons with BMI values of more than 30 roughly doubled in Britain and in the USA during the 80's and 90's. "Well it does appear that our genetic make up does not exactly match our modern living styles and standards. Perhaps God will wake up one day and remodel our genes and bring down our BMI's. But like our other long term government projects, this one is sure going to take time!" state medical experts very philosophically and jovially.

Apart from BMI there are other factions to reckon within the domain of obesity. There is this entity called <u>Central Obesity (or) Visceral Obesity</u>, which is said to be the real culprit in causing damage in obese persons, such as diabetes or heart attack. Sumo wrestlers who look huge and hopelessly obese have surprisingly low visceral obesity, so they escape their share of heart attacks and diabetes, which they would have if they were of the same body weight otherwise. Also their active exercise programmes help reduce the risk of heart attacks which sedentary obese patients tend to have.

There are still other factors in weight gain that seem to

matter. If one gains weight after the age of 18 to 20 years, one is at a greater risk of heart attacks and diabetes. So too is the rate of gain important—anything more than 10 kilos or more than one kilos per year means more trouble.

Modern observations on obesity being a health hazard are matched by the grand old master of scientific medicine, Hippocrates who said, 'Sudden death is more common in those who are naturally fat than in the lean.' So it is an important observation—made both in old and in new age—that obese people die sooner than others.

If mankind is getting obese and if obesity is linked to death than how is longevity increasing? Maybe an interesting question. Obesity epidemic is somewhat recent and will take time to show its bad effects. Currently the increasing longevity is probably due to our improved handling of heart attacks and other related coronary artery diseases, and also the better control of infectious diseases that used to claim lives in the past. It is possible that there are other mischief areas in obese persons like diabetes, hypertension, with resultant kidney damage, eye damage and so on to reckon with. It is also possible that obesity takes 15-20 years to show up as diabetes and another 15 years to play other kinds of mischief. Hence, the *Lancet Medical Journal* mentions it as a time bomb that is ticking away.

Another important observation is that despite the steady increase in obesity in the general population it is not exactly in fashion anywhere in the world. When the average body weights of Miss America contestants were studied and compared to that of other countries such observation came to light.

Overcoming obesity or overweight needs a clear perception. The golden rule to remember is: <u>Obesity is a Medical Problem; not a Cosmetic Problem.</u>

Unfortunately obesity is taken to be a cosmetic problem and not a medical one, which it is. Once this point becomes clear the diet, exercise and lifestyle modifications can help in obesity treatment.

Losings Weight— Some Useful Tips.

1. A sound programme based on shared activity can help a person lose weight faster than just diets.

2. By sharing exercise with a friend four times a week, both recreational fun type activities and intentional weight training and aerobics, the results of weight loss are there to see.

3. Helping a family member lose weight only works if the person concerned (i.e., the obese overweight person) and the person (interested in helping him out) are both committed to honest and open communication. The person who has to lose weight should ask for advice and suggestions enthusiastically.

4. The best diets are not really diets at all—just-healthy foods and conscious eating, only lifestyle change works.

5. When weight loss becomes a shared activity between two members both should have goals, like cutting back on sweets, fried foods, junk foods, etc., and both should support each other in such targets.

6. When two members are sharing a weight loss activity— one who needs the actual weight loss and the other just helping him out, the helper must be a 'friend' first, and a weight loss coach later. Overweight individuals are very sensitive about the weight they have been gaining. They should be approached with care and support, not with a rule book and stick.

7. Compulsive overeating can often mask emotional problems that need to be cleared up with family, friends,

and co-workers. One should get to the root of one's issues and not let unchecked eating be a distraction to the real work that needs to be done. If the problem continues for several months, a doctor's help must be taken.

8. High sodium food will make one retain water for a short time, which is an undesirable bloat if one is managing one's weight. Always check the food. Examples of high sodium food are frozen pizza slices with 1000 mg/slice medium sodium content and be margarine with 120 mg/tsp. A low sodium is fruit with 2-5 mg/entire piece. Doctors recommend about 1500 mg/day of sodium for people who need to cut back.

31

Drugs, Foods and Moods

ARE YOU A PEAR or an APPLE?

What is more dangerous than obesity or general overweight? It is the fat, flab around the abdomen! This increases the risk of heart attack by six times! Generally if the fat is more on the upper aspects of body it is called 'Apple' type and if the fat is more on thigh, buttocks and on lower aspects of the body it is called pear type. The body gets classified as apple-shaped or pear-shaped.

Apple type fat is seen more in Asians; this increases TGL

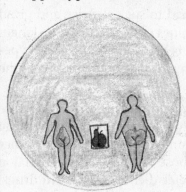

in blood; increases the chances of diabetes and hypertension and also decreases good cholesterol (HDL) in blood.

Women should maintain their waist circumference at 80 cm and men at 90 cm. Never should these limits be crossed. This needs exercise and proper diet. Fatty food ought to be avoided. Our aim is to live long, not have long waistlines!

For many with bulging stomachs and straining waistbands the only dream is to shed the kilos. As waistlines balloon, so do the related health problems. In urban areas the incidence of heart disease has doubled in the past 30 years and experts predict that by the end of year 2005 every fifth diabetic in the world will be an Indian!

Doctors use the BMI (as it is the only reliable tool) to judge whether a patient is overweight. It is calculated (we all know) by taking into account the weight and height of the person. With too much food, too little exercise and modern lifestyle changes which favour gaining weight, more and more Indians are reaching this mark of 25 to 29.9 BMI which groups him as overweight and 30 BMI is pure obesity.

Clearly something must be done to avert the health crisis. But losing weight the 'traditional' way is an uphill task. We all agree on this fact. Nearly all dieters regain the weight they lose. Other methods such as liposuction and stomach stapling can be uncomfortable and dangerous. 'Metabolic Specialists' working in Western countries attribute lifestyle as the main causative factor. Obesity is often lifetime related. Problems of obesity stems from the fact that cooking methods have changed.

When we were young, we had to soak the rice and grind it everyday. Now we have machines to do it—so we no longer burn the calories. Since obesity is also linked to certain types of cancer doctors are using drugs to help patients out of the 'danger zone'.

Doctors widely use two drugs to fight obesity. They are Reductil and Xenical. Some doctors feel that there is no reason to avoid using drugs in the treatment of obesity. Sometimes they can be very useful, argue those doctors. Another section of very conservative doctors prefer diet, exercise. No drugs, they say. Slow and steady means of diet and exercise coupled with lifestyle modifications will win the race of weight reduction.

The Reductil pill (so widely used in urban medical practice) increases the speed at which the body feels full, thus discouraging the patient from eating much. Patients who take the drug lose around 8 per cent of their weight in two years. Xenical stops the fat in the food from being stored in the body. However, the drugs are far from perfect. The problem with Reductil is that it suppresses metabolism. The side effects of xenical are unpleasant. Unabsorbed fat passes with the faeces leading to diarrhoea and sometimes mild incontinence.

The ideal drug would be one that stimulates metabolism while decreasing appetite. We need drugs that amplify normal metabolism and stimulate metabolic rate. This would produce heat instead of the type of energy that the body can turn to fat. One drug that might work in this way is Famoxin, produced by the French Company Grenset. It is still in the trial stages. But early results look promising. Famoxin stimulates the burning of fat and it probably regulates appetite as well. If it works in human trials it could be very useful.

The man-made form of a naturally occurring hormone, Famoxin discourages the body from accumulating fat and promotes the production of heat. Research indicates that a hormone similar to Famoxin is often deficient in obese people. Replacement of this hormone could be getting to the root of the problem. A therapy of this kind should work longer with fewer side effects.

Metabolic stimulants would be useful. It would be like popping an exercise pill—we could eat what we want and the drug would do the exercise for us. Doctors working in urban areas often envisage the discovery of such pills so that they can treat their patients (with obesity) to their full satisfaction. At present most of the doctors feel that drugs may not provide a long-term solution. Change in lifestyles and eating habits plus more and more exercise alone can help fight obesity. Exercise is the most effective weapon against obesity whether it is urban or rural scenario, reiterate health experts.

Facts about our Daily Bread

For more than a decade, health conscious consumers have been chewing down on many low fat oatmeal pancakes and pieces of 12 grain bread. They were motivated by a steady drum beat of good news studies that found that wholegrains that include the bran, the germ and the endosperm protect against a number of diseases and the undeniable fact that valuable nutrients and fibre disappear when grains are refined.

But a growing number of nutritionists, obesity researchers and consumers, annoyed by their seemingly intractable extra pounds, are taking a second look at the once sacrosanct wholegrains. In this age of soaring rates of type 2 diabetes and obesity we all need to limit our consumption of grains— even whole grains—say the new research reports.

· This backlash against wholegrains is yet another nutritional pendulum swing, this time away from fat phobic wholegrain centric diets that did not solve many of the weight problems. 'People forgot that fat free does not mean calorie free' say nutrition experts.

Only 10,000 years ago, a mere evolutionary Blip in the 2.2 million years that humans have been on earth, the main sources of carbohydrates were vegetables and fruits, not grains. We have had very little evolutionary fault wholegrains on other fronts. For example, fibre rich wholegrains contain phytate which inhibits the absorption of minerals including zinc, iron, calcium. But the amount of wholegrain fibre eaten on average by us doesn't warrant us to worry about phytate. Lots of people are still taking such low levels of fibres that constipation and piles have become their companions. With such as situation 'phytate' hardly posses a threat. Unrefined or minimally refined cereals if taken in very large amounts can cause zinc or iron deficiencies, but not in the levels we take. Nutrition experts recommend that overweight people cut back on grains to help reduce their calorie intake; wholegrains must be in moderation because they contain beneficial fibre and disease fighting nutrients.

In 1997 the US food and drug administration acknowledged the cholesterol lowering ability of the soluble fibre from whole oats by allowing label that said that they 'may reduce the risk of heart disease'. In 1999 US FDA went further, allowing products that contain atleast 51 per cent whole grain to carry a label that says they may protect against heart disease and some cancers. The FDA was reacting to the overwhelming evidence that wholegrains protect against disease as do fruits and vegetables. Both vegetables/fruits and wholegrains are healthy foods. They should not be in competition with each other.

Now even the 'new generation dietitians' and modern nutritionists along with health-conscious consumers have started to debate on the relative merits of wholegrains, fruits, vegetables. The Americans still stick to the widely denounced highly processed foods. In fact, fresh fruits, vegetables, wholegrains are among those rare foods that even notoriously over indulgent Americans show no sign of overeating.

Foods and Moods

The foods a person eats can have a huge impact on his need and his energy. A recent study showed 80 per cent of people who cut back on mood suppressors and filled up with mood supporters reported improved mental health, including fewer mood swings, panic attacks, anxiety, less depression. The kind of food we eat is instrumental in endowing in us qualities such as a sense of well being, concentration, alertness, and different energy levels.

There are some chemicals in the brain called the neuron transmitters. Certain neuron transmitters excite and some calm. three chemical neuron transmitters are made in the brain from by products of the food we eat. These are dopamine, norepinephrine, serotonin.

Dopamine and norepinephrine are the alertness chemicals. When the brain is producing these, there is a tendency to think and react more quickly and feel more motivated, attentive and mentally energetic. We have all heard of the term 'adrenaline rush'. Adrenaline also known as epinephrine is in the same family of chemical neurotransmitters. Serotonin is the calming and relaxing chemical. Lab studies show that when the brain is using serotonin, feelings of tension and stress decrease and the mind can concentrate and focus better. Serotonin also reduces the reaction time and depending on the time of day one may feel sleepy or sluggish.

Ayurveda have been explains the connection between moods and foods since long ago. They classified foods into.

1) **Sattvic foods**: Foods like cereals, pulses, sprouts, honey, fruits and vegetables come under this group. These foods keep the mind calm and composed.

2) **Rajasic foods**: Foods like coffee, tea, fish, eggs, salt, chocolate. These foods agitate the mind and increase the activity, passion, emotions like jealousy.

3) **Tamasic foods**: This group includes leftovers, alcohol, tobacco, non-vegetarian items. These foods promote indifference, anger, greed, inertia and lethargy.

Now modern science is rediscovering these facts and the connection between the moods and foods. Take a look at these mood supporters and suppressors, say nutritionists.

1. Calming Carbohydrates

Eating carbohydrate makes one feel better less stressed and calm as the energy is up. However, all carbohydrates are not equal in their ability to offer mood altering results. The best way to consume carbohydrates is as wholegrains and complex carbohydrates. Wholegrains are broken down over a long period of time keeping a constant flow of serotonin in the body. Complex carbohydrates are present in cereals such as rice, wheat, ragi, corn, jowar, potato and dals. Snack food that helps one concentrate better and ward off tension in the middle of the day includes popcorn, baked potato, vegetable sandwiches, and fresh fruits.

2. Peppy Proteins

Protein releases brain chemicals for self esteem, optimism, impulse/appetite control, calm and good feelings and good sleep. If one is feeling sluggish protein encourages the production of dopamine and norepinephrine which produce alertness, mental energy and faster reaction time. The effects of eating protein lasts for about two to three hours. One should not eat proteins in large quantities several hours before bedtime or this will cause difficulties in falling asleep. Proteins also contains amino acids that aid in the creation of endorphins— mood-regulation neurotransmitters. So it is essential for people suffering from stress, depression or anxiety. High protein foods include fish, egg white, sprouts, nuts. Grapes and oranges, even capsicum taken in informed quantity, are helpful.

3. Fruits and Vegetables

Vegetables and fruits colourfully arranged in a market, giving out nice smells, tempting flavours—all these have a calming effect on us. The very sight, the very smell and thought of flavour/taste calms us. Vegetables are loaded with vitamins, minerals, and other nutrients that make good moods possible. Fruits tend to be rich in vitamin B_6 which the brain needs to make serotonin, a neurotransmitter that facilitates happy moods. They are also full of antioxidants, which protect the brain cell membranes. It is recommended to have four to five one-cup servings of fruits and veggies daily. The fresher the produce, the more nutrients one gets.

4. Magic of Water

Our bodies are three-quarters water dehydration makes us feel fuzzy and dull. Most people are dehydrated. We have lost the ability to recognise the thirst. We may eat when we are actually thirsty. We need eight glasses of water (2 litres) every day to replace lost fluids in the body (more so in hot weather and if exercising). This is on top of all other drinks.

5. Caffeine

Most people know about the yo-yo effect caffeine (present in coffee, tea, coca colas) can have on moods—sleepy one minute, giddy the next—but many don't realise the role it has on the overall mental health. Studies have shown that caffeine inhibits the brain levels of serotonin and melatonin, a hormone that affects our sleep cycles as well as depleting vitamin B, vitamin C, potassium, calcium and zinc. These impact sleep quality and duration as well as tolerance to stress. As serotonin levels are suppressed, a tendency to be depressed, irritable, obsessive, worried, or fearful increases.

6. Sweets

Anybody looking for a radical change in his/her moods must drop processed sugar. Sugar or sweet temporarily lifts the mood but the insulin rush that happens after eating the sweet, rapidly brings down both the sugar and the mood.

7. Alcohol

Has a sedative effect in small quantities. However chances of misusing alcohol are quite high. Moreover, the long-term use of alcohol may have negative effects like liver diseases, cancer, brain cell loss and diabetes. Although alcohol can lift moods its other effects make it a poor choice as a mood lifter.

8. Food Deprivation

Depriving oneself of food can also mess up moods. The person gets depressed, irritable, one's doesn't have the energy to exercise. All the vital nutrients are also missed. There will be weight loss—then gain back—all leading to low self-esteem.

32

Small Kids, Big Problem

As a fall out of obesity children now battle a host of diseases usually found in adults. Sedentary lifestyles and changed eating habits may lead to a health catastrophe among them.

More and more youngsters are falling prey to obesity and most have no idea how to stay healthy. Neither do their parents if one goes by case studies. Parents start worrying only when children turn 15 or 16. Otherwise they think that the chubbier the kids, the healthier; they call them cute, say dietetians. Doctors and health care professionals warn of a health catastrophe if the fast increasing number of overweight children is not brought down. The figures are alarming. The Nutrition Foundation of India which examined 4,300 children of middle and upper middle class families in Delhi found 26 per cent of them overweight and 3.9 per cent plain obese. The All India Institute of Medical Sciences, Delhi, warns that the death rate will shoot up to 33 per cent (from the present 9 per cent) especially among the youth, on account of non-communicable diseases like heart problems caused by obesity. The situation is the same everywhere a study by the Subharti Medical College, in Meerut, Uttar Pradesh among 1,500 students showed that 9 per cent of them were obese. The College of Home Science, Mumbai, has found that more girls are overweight and obese (65 per cent) than boys.

In fact NFI points out that nearly a third of men and more than half the women in the upper middle class in India are overweight, a figure that can drastically increase if the problem is not tackled in childhood. Nearly 30 per cent of all obese adults were obese as children.

As we discussed in an earlier section it is ironic that we have problems at two extreme ends of the spectrum. Undernourished children on one side then an opposite kind of problem on the other side—that of excessive nutrition.

Many believe that hormonal imbalances are the main reasons why kids are plump but that is a very minute percentage, say paediatricians.

Junk food is linked to violent behaviour

- The next time a person throws a plate at you or stamps angrily on something don't blame him for his violent behaviour. The violence could actually be sparked by his nutritionally drab diet, according to some scientists. They argue that giving violent young offenders a cocktail of mineral, vitamins, fatty acids seems to transform a pit-bull-like kid into a double poodle type. (Our *Bhagavad Gita* has already stated that *tamasic* food causes delusional darkness of mind.)

- Many studies state that adding nutrients to the inmate's diet (in offenders' homes) remarkably reduces antisocial behaviour.

- Avoid junk food for yet an other reason!

It is the lifestyle and the environment one grows up in that matter more. After school, kids used to play out in the field but today they go for the TV remote control or internet browsing. Aggravating the problem is the documented fact that when children watch TV they snack more, often on unhealthy junk foods that are high in salt and calories and low in fibre. An average Indian does not have much information about nutrition. We equate our health with weight.

This means a double whammy. With more parents working the already sedentary children (parents in Indian metros feel their children are softer if they stay home and watch TV or computer when the parents are out) are eating the kind of food that adds generously to their adipose tissues. Besides, children whose both parents were obese were more likely to be obese.

It is not junk food alone that adds to the lard. Even in traditional cooking, refined wheat and polished rice have displaced wholegrain as the staple cereal. Even traditional nutritious delicacies can turn into a fattener, *e.g., Gajar ka halwa* is a good source of beta carotene when cooked in milk but in most sweet meat stalls, it is now prepared in calorie-rich ghee!

School timings in big cities are also to blame for unhealthy eating. In Delhi, classes often begin at 7.30 a.m. and are over by noon, ostensibly to help the public transport system cope better with the morning rush hour. But this has played havoc with children's routines. Most children leave for school at around 6.30 a.m. Many do not have breakfast and do not bring lunch either, say many teachers and nutrition experts doing community studies. So the net result is they end up eating junk food from canteens.

While a few elite schools provide wholesome meals to students most have canteens that are part sponsored by soft drink giants or fast food chains. Delhi government issues circulars to city schools to ban junk food and to provide nutritious food in canteens; however, the situation never improves!

Recent studies by doctors at the paediatric department of the Post-Graduate Institute, Chandigarh, revealed that decreased outdoor activity, prolonged TV viewing and family histories were all associated with obesity. There could also be clinical reasons behind the rising incidence of obesity in India.

Syndrome X or dysmetabolic syndrome is present more in Indians than foreigners. It is a defective gene action, where the body insulin action is not adequate and so adipose tissue is not broken down. Obesity is not a separate entity but a metabolic component of syndrome X comprising diabetes, lipid disorders, cardiovascular disease and high BP.

The children with that "little extra flab" can develop a host of deadly diseases later on. Obesity is an independent risk factor for cardiovascular diseases, diabetes, arthritis.

Some recent surveys showed that 35 per cent of Delhi school children had vision problems and 40 per cent had dental problems. These problems are caused by unbalanced diets and excessive addition to TV and computers.

Doctors say that the warning signs are already showing up. Today there are instances of adolescents with type II diabetes (a lifestyle disease found in adults), more and more teens are developing high BP, high cholesterol and conditions preceding diabetes.

Tailor-made weight loss programmes are available for children in fitness centres. Counselling the parents and kids is a major component of these programmes. Usually a normal programme lasts two and half months. Medical history of kids and their eating habits are both studied. Usually the 'wrong' eating habits is the culprit for the children being fat, say, majority of fitness experts.

Many children are taking the matter seriously. 'Being motivated' is the main requisite. Bariatric surgery, which cuts down adipose tissue is slowly becoming popular in India.

Certain hospitals are working on methods of reducing fat using electrodes. The idea is to make the person eat less by creating artificial impulses from the stomach to a pacemaker in the brain signalling that the stomach is full. Another method is cutting short the large intestine so that fat absorption is reduced. However, this leads to less minerals being absorbed. Hence it is not recommended for growing children, except in cases of morbid obesity.

Preoccupied with combating malnutrition the government has paid little attention to the problem if obesity. The programmes on nutrition in the tenth five-year plan focus entirely on under-nutrition and efforts to achieve optimal levels of nutrition. Besides Indians by and large do not accept obesity as a problem. Parents have to be convinced that their kids are fat and need to reduce weight. This is a 'big' difficulty, as most of the parents don't agree. Psychologically too, being fat exacts a big price from a growing child—a loss of self-confidence. Living in an image-conscious world these kids easily fall prey to depression. Studies in the USA have proved that fat children are unhappier than others. A little effort from schools and parents could go a long way in solving what health care professionals call 'an economic disaster waiting to happen' in health care costs. Better food, more physical activity, regulated TV habits, education about healthy living in schools—all these are the need of the hour. The best example is Singapore. Obesity in the city state's kids shot up from 2 per cent in the late 70's to 17 per cent by 1992 forcing the health promotion board to take up a massive compaign. Teachers were trained (with schools being the main target of compassing) to impart better eating habits to the kids, modification of the foods available at school canteens and promotion of lifestyle with physical exercise— these three steps bought fantastic results! Obesity fell to less than 10 per cent by 1998.

It is time the next generation wakes up and sweats it out, lest India should go the US way: obesity has been declared an epidemic there!

CHILDHOOD OBESITY

Limit or cutout junk foods.

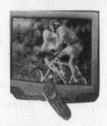

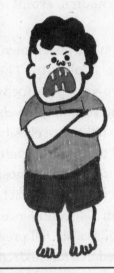

RESTRICT sedentary TV watching and encourage correct eating habits, balanced diet and physical activity.

Instructions and Information for Parents/Kids

1. Adipose Barrier: Fat accumulates in a person's body when the input energy (essentially the food and drink we take in) is in excess of the output. A body uses energy primarily for three things: (1) Resting, (2) Thermogenic processes such as digesting, (3) Physical activities.

    Children need energy for growth too. The energy spent through exertion varies massively from person to person and determines whether a person is fat or not. If the intake of food (energy) is more the balance is stored as fat (adipose tissue). For children also obesity is assessed by BMI.

    BMI over 25 kg/m^2—overweight child.

    BMI over 30 kg/m^2—obese child.

    For children the situation could be worse. In obese children not only is the quantity of fat in each cell higher but the number of fat cells is also three to four times more than in non obese children.

2. What should the children eat and how much should they gain?

1) One banana: 114 calories.

2) French-fries (small serving): 210 calories.

3) Thin crust pizza: 255 calories.

4) Hamburger: 330 calories.

5) Chicken sandwich: 710 calories.

6) One cup rice: 170 calories.

7) Dal makhani: 196 calories.

One must carefully monitor what the children eat. The aim should be right food, right quantities; junk food to be restricted or chucked out completely.

3. Fitness trainers say that the number of obese and overweight children coming in for weight reduction programmes are on the rise.

Obesity in Kids

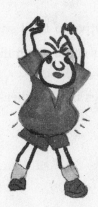 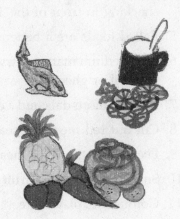

Some Tips

1. Salads are good.

2. Cut out red meat; and seafood can be tried.

3. Milk shakes are healthy substitutes for colas.

4. Fruits and vegetables must be included in diet.

They are put through a circuit-training programme which involves exercising all body parts. To lose all the flab accumulated by eating, sleeping and watching TV one needs some intensive weight reduction programme. If the family members have high BP or diabetes related to obesity, children should be encouraged more so to lose the flab so that those diseases don't bother them. Strict diet of vegetable soup and fruits must be given, and chocolates, soft drinks, etc., to be completely banned.

4. Lifestyle measures to combat obesity in kids:

   1. Limit time spent in front of the TV.

   2. Eat healthy food—try salads and clear soups.

   3. Order better at fast food outlets—a pizza is a better alternative to a burger and a mildshake to a cola.

   4. Have an early home-cooked dinner. This reduces snacking in front of the TV.

   5. Baked foods are a better alternative to fried stuff.

   6. The medium matters—try sweets cooked in milk rather than oil or ghee.

   7. Include more dals and vegetables in your diet.

   8. Cut out red meat; try seafood.

   9. Fix regular times for meals.

   10. Snack on fruits and fruit juices.

   11. Go outside; play more.

       a. Try jogging at least two or three times a week.

       b. Cycling is also a good option.

   12. Do not try fad dieting.

Parents, teachers or fitness experts can only guide the kids but the initiative and motivation should come from kids. Today's kids are very intelligent. What they need is correct guidance and ideal role models. Parents and teachers should play these roles and the results will be excellent, for everybody to see.

33

Some Astonishing Data

(With reference to obesity, overweight and underweight, the following facts are gleaned from the Guinness Book of World Records and Limca Book of Records.)

Weight Records

'Lightest' Humans

The *highest* recorded adult was Lucia Zarate born in San Carlos, Mexico on January 2, 1863. At birth she weighed 2 ½ lbs. This emaciated Ateliotic dwarf of 26 ½ inches weighed 4.4 lbs at the age of 17. She fattened up to 13 lbs by her 20th birthday. She died in October 1889.

The thinnest recorded adults of normal height are those suffering from Simmonds disease (Hypophyzeal Cachexia). Losses up to 65 per cent of the original body weight have been recorded in females, with a 'low' of 45 lbs in the case of Emma Shaller (1868-1890) of St. Louis Missour, who stood 5 feet 2-inches tall. In cases of anorexia nervosa, a weight of under 10-lbs has been reported.

It was recorded that the American exhibitionist, Rosa Lee Plemons (born 1873), weighed 27 lbs at the age of 18. Edward C. Hogner (1892-1962), alias Eddie Masher, is alleged to have weighed only 48 lbs at a height of 5 feet 7 inches. He was also known as the 'skeleton dude'. In August 1825, the biceps measurement of Cloude Ambroise Sevrat (born April 10, 1797, died April 6, 1826) of Troyes, France, was 4 inches and the distance between his back and his chest was less than 3 inches. He stood 5 feet 7 ½ inches and weighed 78 lbs but in another account was described as 5 feet 4 inches and only 36 lbs.

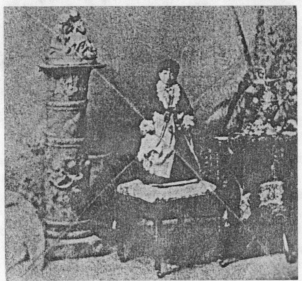

LIGHTEST HUMAN ADULT: Lucia Zarate of Mexico weighed 4.7 lbs. at the age of 17 and stood 26½ inches tall. At birth in 1863, she weighed 2½ lbs.

Heaviest Man

The heaviest medically weighed human was the 6 feet ½ inches tall Robert Earl Hughes (born 1926) of Monticello, Illinois. An 11 ¼ baby, he weighed

203 lbs at 6 years

378 lbs at 10 years

546 lbs at 13 years

693 lbs at 18 years

896 lbs at 25 years

945 lbs at 27 years

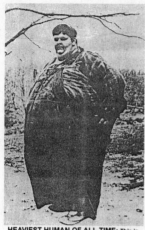

HEAVIEST HUMAN OF ALL TIME: This is Robert Earl Hughes when he weighed only 700 lbs. He later reached a top weight of 1,069 lbs. He was buried in a coffin the size of a piano case.

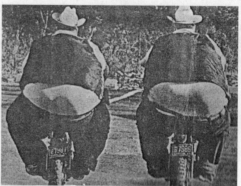

HEAVIEST TWINS: The McCreary brothers, Bill and Ben, weighed 660 and 640 lbs., left and right respectively,in 1970.They now tag wrestle under the names Billy and Benny McGuire at over 700 lbs. each.

His greatest record has been the weight recorded in February, 1958. It was 1,069 lbs. He weighed 1,041 lbs at the time of his death. His claimed waist of 122 inches, his chest of 124 inches and his upper arms of 40 inches were the greatest on record. Hughes died of uremia (condition caused by retention of urinary matter in the blood) in a trailer at Bremen, Indiana, on July 10, 1958, aged 32, and was buried in Benville cemetery, near Mount Sterling, Illinois. His coffin as large as a Piano case measuring 7 feat by 4 feet 4 inches and weighing more than 1,100 lbs and had to be lowered by a crane. It was once claimed by a commercial interest that Hughes had weighed 1,500 lbs 40 per cent exaggeration.

The only other men for whom weights of 800 lbs or more have been reliably reported are listed below:

1. Mills Darden (1798 -1857), U.S. (7 ft 6 in), 1,020 lbs

2. John Hansan Craig (1856-94), U.S. (6 ft 5 inch), 907 lbs

3. Arthur Knorr (1914-60), U.S (6 ft. 1 inch), 900 lbs

4. Toubi (born 1946), Cameroon, 857 ½ lbs

5. T.A Valenzuela (1895-1937), Mexico (5 ft 11 inch), 850 lbs

6. David Maguire (1904-1935), U.S. (5 ft 10 inch), 810 lbs

7. William J. Cobb (born 1926), U.S (6 ft 0 inch), 802 lbs

8. Unnamed patient (born 1936-1973), Richmond Virginia, 800 ¼ lbs

a. gained 300 lbs in the last 6 months of his life.

b. reduced to 232 lbs by July 1965.

c. won $ 1,000 in a 'bonny baby' contest in New York in 1858.

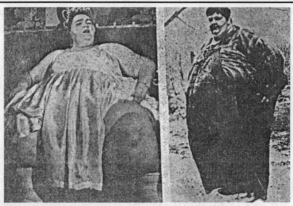

HEAVIEST WOMAN (left): Mrs Percy Pearl
Washington could have weighed as much as 880 lbs
Robert Earl Hughes, once weighed at exactly 1069 lbs,
tipped the scales at 203 lbs when he was 6 years old.
In this photo he wighed only 700 lbs.

The heaviest human in medical history has been Jon Brower Minnoch (b Sept 29, 1941) of Bainbridge Island, Washington, who was carried on planking by a rescue team into University Hospital, Seattle, in March 1978. Dr. Robert Schwartz, the endocrinological consultant, estimated by extrapolating his intake and elimination rates that he was 'probably more' than 1,400 lb. It took 13 attendants to roll him over in his hospital bed. After nearly 2 years on a 1200-calorie-per-day diet he was discharged at 476 lbs. He had to be readmitted in October 1981 having reportedly gained 200 lbs in 7 days. This former taxicab driver stands 6 ft 1 inch in tall.

Francis John Lang (b 1934), alias Michael Walker of Clinton, Iowa, was attributed a weight of 1,187 lbs. He could not be admitted for treatment for inflammation of the gall bladder to the Veteran's Administration Hospital, Houston, Texas because of the impossibility of getting him through the doors. He was treated in a trailer in the car park and discharged on Jan. 5, 1972 unweighed but estimated to be between 900 and 1,000 lbs. The more precise weight above was claimed for him while he was suffering from drug-induced bulimia, in the summer of 1971 when he was working with the Christian Farms of Killeen, Texas. There is, however, no independent corroboration for the precise upper weight quoted, although photographic evidence suggests the weight was possibly reliable. By Feb. 1980 Lang (6 ft 2 inch) had reduced to 369 lbs.

Heaviest Woman—The heaviest woman ever recorded was the late Mrs. Percy Pearl Washington (born Louisiana, 1926) who died in a hospital in Milwaukee on October 9, 1972. The hospital scales registered only up to 800 lbs, but she was believed to weigh about 880 lbs. The previous weight record for a woman was set 84 years earlier at 850 lbs although an unsubstantiated report exists of a woman, Mrs. Ida Maitland (1892-1932) of Springfield, Mississippi, who had a bust measurement of 152 inches and weighed 911 lbs. She was said to have died trying to pick a four leaf clover.

A more reliable and better documented case was that of Mrs. Flora Mae (or May) Jackson (Née King), a 5-foot-9-inch Negress born in 1930 at Shuqualak, Mississippi. She weighed 10 lbs, at birth: 267 lbs at the age of 11: 621 lbs at 25 and 840 lbs shortly before her death in Meridian, Florida, on December 9, 1965. She was known in show business as "Baby Flo".

Greatest Weight Differential—The greatest weight differential recorded for a married couple is 922 lbs in the case of Mills Darden (1,020 lbs.) of North Carolina and his wife Mary (98 lbs.) Despite her diminutiveness, however, Mrs. Darden bore her husband three children before her death in 1837.

Slimming

The greatest recorded slimming feat was that of William J. Cobb (born 1926) alias "Happy Humphrey" a professional wrestler of Macon, Georgia. It was reported in July 1965 that he had reduced fron 802 lbs to 232 lbs, a loss of 570 lbs in 3 years. His waist measurement declined from 101 inches to 44 inches.

The U.S. circus fat lady, Mrs. Celesta Geyer (born 1901), alias Dolly Dimples, reduced from 553 lbs to 152 lbs in 1950–51, a loss of 401 lbs in 14 months. Her vital statistics diminished *pan passu* from 79–84–84 to a *svelte* 34–28–36. Her book *How I lost 400 lbs* was not a bestseller. In December 1967 she was reportedly down to 110 lbs.

SLIMMING SPEED CHAMP: Paul Kimelman lost 357 lbs in 8 months when he was 21. Before he went on a crash diet he weighed 487 lbs. The result—130 lbs. He now remains slim at 175 lbs.

Heaviest Twins

The heaviest twins were the performers Billy Leon and Benny Loyd MeCary, alias Billy and Benny Mc Guire (b Dec. 7, 1946) of Henderson-vile, NC. In Nov, 1978, they were weighed at 743 lbs (Billy) and 723 lbs (Benny) and had 84-in waists. Billy died of heart failure on July 13, 1979, in Niagara Falls, Canada, after falling from his mini-bike. He was buried in a square coffin with a total weight of over 1,000 lbs in Hendersonville. A hydraulic lift was needed to lower the coffin to its final

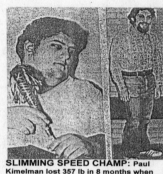

SLIMMING SPEED CHAMP: Paul Kimelman lost 357 lb in 8 months when he was sult—130 lbs. He now remains slim at 175 lbs.

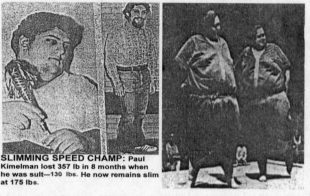

HEAVIEST TWINS: Billy 2nd Benny McCrary, with 84-in waists more than 700 lbs when they were tag-team wrestlers.

resting place. After one 6-week slimming course in a hospital, they emerged weighing 5 lbs more each.

Heaviest Boy (Limca Book of Records 1992)

Nine-year-old Gajanan Shiv Shankar Kacharde of Dhanki village in the Yeotmal district of Maharashtra weighs an incredible 87 kg. He is presently undergoing treatment.

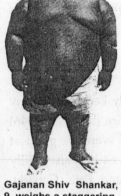

Gajanan Shiv Shankar, 9, weighs a staggering 87 kg.

Slimming

Those currently struggling and starving to lose weight, may find this a little hard to believe. But 26-year-old Vijay Udani, a chartered accountant by profession has certainly proved a point and created a record simultaneously. Prior to April 1988, the 6 ft Udani weighed 142 kg and was excessively overweight. But by December 1988, he had lost 50 kg. This was achieved by a walking and jogging regimen for over 12 km, 7 days a week, Diet was strictly vegetarian and restricted to one main meal a day supplemented by milk and curd. From December onwards, the dieting was discontinued, but the exercise kept up, now 5 times a week. He managed to lose a further 12 kg from January 1989 to December 1989 without dieting but continuing the exercise routine. He now weighs 80 kgs and has lost 21 inches on the waist and 24 inches on the hips. He is trim, fit and full of confidence.

.... **Slimming** ....

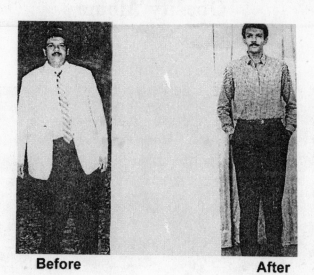

Before   **After**

34

Obesity Album

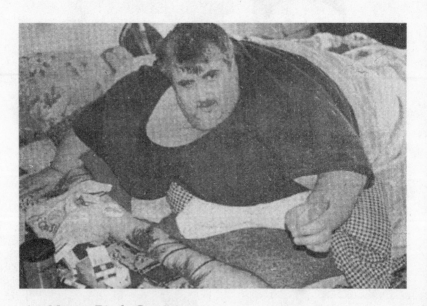

1. Name: Risab Corsigian

    Weight: 300 kgs

    Resides in Turkey

    Profession: Icecream seller

    Literally a 'flesh mountain'. He consumes 'large large' quantities of food every day. Doctors have advised a gastric bypass surgery for him, otherwise he will be a victim to the deadly clutches of obesity.

2. 'JUMBO'—Dictionary describes this word as a very large thing, e.g., jumbo jet—large jet aircraft.

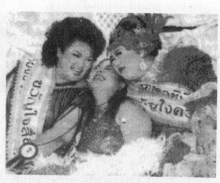

So what does the picture here has to do with all this? The picture depicts the winners of 'Jumbo queen contest' which selects the winners on the basis of their overweight! The larger you are the better are your chances of becoming the jumbo queen.

3. Both these students belong to the same class, same school Both belong to Malaysia.

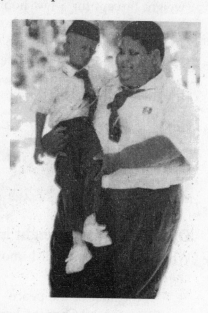

Small Person

Name: Mohammed Mauz

Age: 15

Ht: 3 ½ Feet.

Wt: 14 kg

Large Person

Name: Mohmmed Anoor

Age: 14

Ht : 5 ¼ feet.

Wt : 140 kg !

Obesity and Overweight in Comic Strips

When it comes to comic strips Two Too Fat characters come to our mind immediately.

1. Laurel and Hardy— This combination of comic characters, 'one fat and one slim' makes a perfect pair.

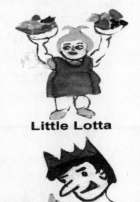

Obesity & overweight in comic strips

2. Little Lotta

Who comes is Richie Rich comics. So fat and so adorable.

Read this witty strip from Archie. Nobody can forget Jughead Jones when one mentions food. Isn't it amazing that he eats and eats but never puts on weight (except for a few hours after a heavy meal)? The 'metabolism' of Jughead Jones needs some detailed study. "His voracious appetite and lean body" are every fitness aspirant's dream.

Little Lotta

Jughead

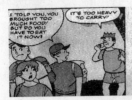

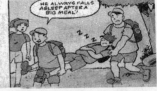

Obesity and Overweight in Movies

When it comes to English movies I can remember two obese characters:

1. 'The villain of the peace' who always comes in between (very rudely) Charlie Chaplin and his girlfriend. That huge figure, evil eyes and the expression on the face when

Charlie Chaplin annoys him (the usual stamping of his feet), it is so hilarious!

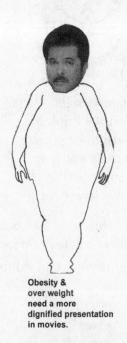

Obesity &
over weight
need a more
dignified presentation
in movies.

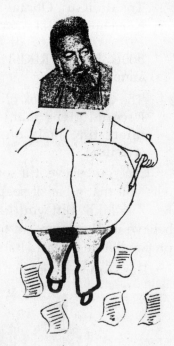

2. Eddie Murphy in *Nutty Professor*

When it comes to our Indian movies my earliest memory of an obese overweight character is that of Asit Sen in *Jagriti*. The lovable Tun Tun, Preeti Ganguly (*in Khatta Meeta*), not to forget that vovacious eater in *Bombay to Goa*.

In the recent times Mohanlal in the Malayalam movie *Uncle Bun*, and Anil Kapoor in the Hindi movie *Badhai Ho Badhai*.

Sumo Wrestling

1. The sport's origins in Japan certainly date from c 23 BC. The heaviest ever Sumotori is Kazuhisa Shiki alias Genkaiho (named Rinho) who in 1981 at a height of 5 ft 9 ½ inches attained 447.6 lbs weight, amassed by overeating a high protein stew called *Chankonale*.

2. Yokozuna refers to grand champion in sumo wrestling.

3. Toshimitsu Obata (alias Kitanomi) has set a record in 1978 winning 82 of the 90 bouts that top RIKISHI fight annually.

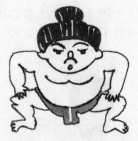

4. The Guinness Book of World Records gives many such interesting facts on sumo wrestling.

The overweight sports. When we think of overweight or obesity we can't but help remembering sumo wrestlers.

Can you believe it if someone tells you that a bar of soap costs Rs. 7 ½ lakh. But you have to believe it. This is not an ordinary soap. This soap has been prepared from the fat of Italian Prime Minister, Silvio Berluconi.

This soap was kept in a Switzerland museum as an exhibit

This soap costs 7 lakhs!

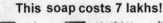

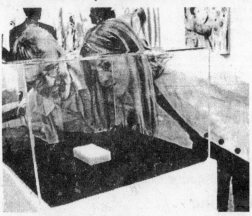

THE
CHERISHED
FAT

during the year-end exhibition. This extraordinary soap was purchased for Rs. 7 ½ lakh in an auction.

The Italian Prime Minister was operated recently and excess fat was removed from his body. This soap is a product of that removed fat!

'Heavy' Personality Popular

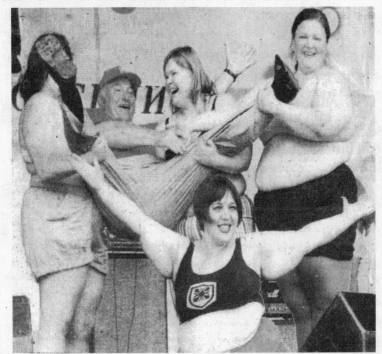

The above picture shows the contestants who took part in a contest conducted in Moscow for overweight women. The 2012 olympic games are going to be held in Russia, and this contest was organised to mark this great event.

When we think of popular personalities who were heavy set and big in appearance one name flashes in mind immediately—the famous English writer Ernest Hemingway.

He made a humble start but then became a force to be reckoned with in modern writing. In 1954 he was awarded the Nobel Prize for literature for his narrative art as shown in his famous book *The Old Man and the Sea*. His life long interest included fishing, shooting, skiing and bull-ring since boyhood. He had a huge, heavy, bulky appearance and many of the characters in his works had such an appearance. He was bulky, and enormous in bearing, and this reflected as the 'look' for many of his characters.

Fedrick Duel—The 'flesh mountain' of America. A year back his weight was 1,072 pounds. When he had to be taken to the hospital his bedroom wall had to be broken. After four months this was the first time he came out of his bedroom confinement. The 43-year-old Fedrick could not sit, turn about while sleeping plus suffered from heart disease and diabetes.

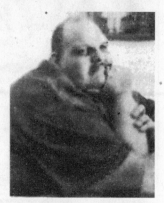

He got operated in the hospital for his heart condition and has now lost 573 lbs in these last 12 months. That is to say, his weight has become half of his original weight in one year.

573 lbs gone in one year

"Big Baby"

A woman in Brazil gave birth to a baby weighing 8 kg. Usually a healthy mother gives birth to a baby weighing 2 ½ to 3 ½ kg and such babies grow well. But this 8 kg baby born to the Brazilian woman <u>Fransisco</u> (aged 38) could be removed only by a surgery from the mother's womb. Both the mother and baby are fine, say doctors.

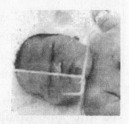

The baby has been nicknamed 'Big baby'. The mother was

suffering from diabetes and hence such a big baby, reason doctors. This baby has the unique distinction of being the heaviest baby born so far in Brazil. The baby was infused with IV glucose to maintain blood sugar level.

Celebrities on Diets

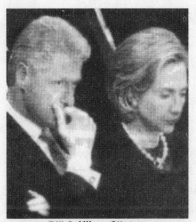

Bill & Hilary Clinton

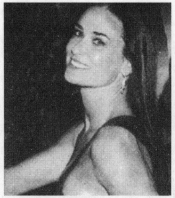

Demi Moore

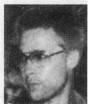

Brad Pitt

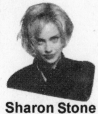

Sharon Stone

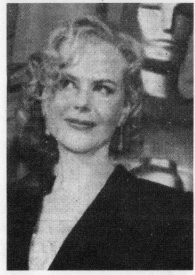

Rene Zellweger

1. Geri Halliwell, Minnie Drivo, Sarah Jessica Parker have tried the Atkins Nutritional Approach Diet.

2. Bill and Hilary Clinton vouch for the Sooth Beach plan.

3. Jennifer Aniston, Brad Pitt, Matthew Perry, Rene Zellweger, Cindy Crawford, Demi Moore, and Sandra Bullock applaud the Zone.

4. Tori Spelling and Sharon Stone talk highly about the Sugar Busters diet.

Kathakali

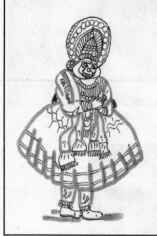

When we see the Kathakali dance of Kerala we often wonder at the appearance of the dancer. The dancer looks obese and overweight. His costume and attire are designed in such a way that it makes him look overweight. It is not the dancer, but it is his garb and makeup that make him appear overweight. It is a 'pseudo overweight' look. The movements and steps of the dancer are very graceful in the Katha Kali dance a unique dance form of Kerala, south India.

35

Obesity in Hindu Mythology and Fairy Tales

Obesity and Overweight in Hindu Mythology

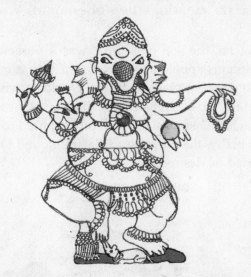

The mouth-watering delicious modaka in the hand represents the presence of a 'Supreme Principle' within the 'space'. It is not to be interpreted as a food item.

1. Ganapati, the celebrated elephant god, is often portrayed as a fat, obese pot bellied god. One must remember that this 'form' has deep, significant, inner meaning. The word

'Brahma' has many meanings. One of its meaning is 'huge, all pervading' God or who has everything contained within him. He is omnipresent and omnipotent. He is pervading in every aspect, be it the huge sky or the massive earth. To symbolise this concept 'Ganapati' is portrayed as elephant-faced and big-bellied.

2. Though Lord Krishna was fat, chubby and cuddly (thanks to all the butter) in his childhood, as he grew into his teens and adulthood he achieved a trim, fit and agile body. This very well signifies the importance of shedding the baby fat and becoming slim and trim.

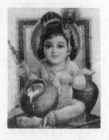

Mahabharata mentions two obese and overweight characters:

1. Ghatotkacha, the son of Bhima, was a voracious eater. His gluttonous appetite however came to use in stopping a marriage taking place against the bride's wishes. The movie *Maya Bazaar* depicts this hilarious episode where Ghatotkacha consumes all the food prepared to serve the guests. Finally, the children of Balarama and Duryodana get married as desired.

GHATOTKACHA

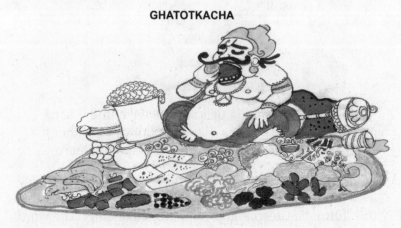

2. In all the epics and *Puranas* male and female demons are
represented as obese, overweight, overeating beasts. The
justification is 'A man is what he eats, how he eats'. The
overeating demons are real beasts. Bakasura, a demon,
had a voracious appetite, not satisfied by huge quantities
of meat, curd, delicacies, rice, intoxicating liquors. He even
ate human beings. Bhima finally killed him and put an
end to his evil deeds.

3. Among the Pandavas Bhima had a voracious appetite.
Kunti would divide the food (while they were in exile) in
two equal portions. One half would go to Bhima, the other
half would be shared by the other brothers and herself.
Bhima being born of the wind had great strength and a
mighty appetite Vrikodara, one of the names of Bhima,
means wolf-bellied—as a wolf always looks famished and
however much it might eat, its hunger is never satisfied.
Bhima had an insatiable hunger.

4. The Akshaya patra (a vessel which held a never failing
supply of food) episode in Mahabharata has great
significance. The explanation is that as the whole universe
is contained in Sri Krishna, his satisfaction with a single
grain of rice satisfied for the time the hunger of all beings
including that of "always angry" says Durvasa.

5. While describing Goddess Parvati most of the shlokas and
chants depict her as one being a delicate, slim, trim, thin
slender and graceful like a creeper (Lata) plant. A perfect
figure—devoid of even a single ounce of unwanted flesh—
is what the 'Devi' has. The statues of the goddess in
temples are based on these facts.

Every year during the festival of lights, Deepavali, in the
holy city of Varanasi, the beautiful idol of Goddess Annapoorni
(the one who provides food to the whole universe) is carried
on a beautiful golden chariot decorated with delicious laddoos.

The goddess with a vessel of food and spoon on her hands sits with a divine radiant smile on her lips. What is the message behind this smile? That she has food for everybody's need but not for their greed. Any excessive appetite, overburdened with food, overfeeding, gluttony or insatiable craving for food is not to be entertained—conveys the sweet smile on her lips.

We have all read about the chakravyuha (unique wheel-like formation) formed by the Kauravas into which the Pandava prince Abhimanyu got caught and killed in the Mahabarata war.

Fruits

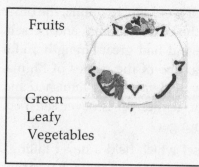

Green
Leafy
Vegetables

The new age chakravyuha to crush obesity & overweight consists of:

- Exercise
- Diet foods
- Giving up fat and sedentary habits.

Obesity needs a similar formation with diet, exercise, and lifestyle modification. This unique combination of fitness programme will crush the overweight and obesity.

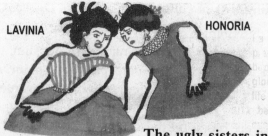

LAVINIA   HONORIA

The ugly sisters in Cinderella

Every story has thin and fat characters.

Take the fairy tales, for example.

1. *Cinderella*: Here the prince was head over heels in love

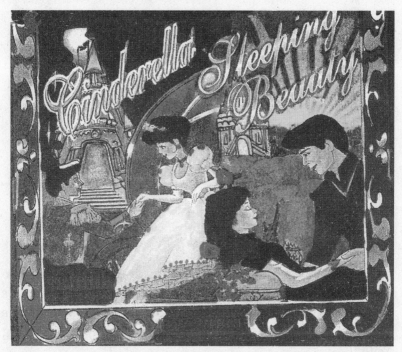

with the slim, trim Cinderella whereas the ugly sisters who were obese and grossly overweight were met with absolute disapproval. They were declared ugly, unfit and grotesque.

2. *Sleeping Beauty*: The handsome her was attracted by the slim and trim beautiful princess who had pricked her finger on the spool of a spinning wheel and was sleeping under the spell of the nasty witch, Ursula. He was so charmed by the 'delicate' princess, he kissed her and she woke up.

36

Latest Developments and Reports

Juice: The Pound Packer

If you are offering beverages like soft drinks or fruit juice to quench your child's thirst, you could be increasing your child's risk of overweight or obesity. Beverages that contain calories can take the blame for weight problems in many of the young patients.

Twenty per cent of the kids who are overweight are so because they consume too many calories. Unlike candies and savouries that people know are fattening when eaten in quantity, families are relatively unaware that beverages are caloric as well.

Health professionals are concerned that children who mindlessly consume artificial fruit juice and soft drinks are jeopardising their health. In the overweight management programmes families come in and don't know why their children are gaining weight because they don't eat that much. The parents (in majority) and their kids do not have any idea how much juice the children are consuming, report the health journals.

There have been cases where one girl had drunk a gallon (3.7 l) of orange juice a day and had gained 31.7 kg over a year. Though this extreme case reported in a foreign country may be an exception, nevertheless it does ring an alarm regarding the seriousness of this problem.

Although fruit juice has nutrients that aren't found in soft drinks, it can still contribute to excess weight gain if children drink too much.

An 8-oz (236 ml) glass of juice is 120 calories. If a person drinks one extra glass a day he can put on 10 lbs. (4.5 kg) a year! Doctors recommend that kids have to run a mile a day to burn off the juice, not even to lose weight! It is a matter of concern that parents are giving juice to infants! There is no need to give infants juice before six months. If infants and young children are given sweetened drinks to satisfy their thirst (fruit juice's natural sugars provide the sweet taste), it can create a habit.

Offering infants juice before solid foods could risk their having juice replace breast milk or infant formula in the diet. This can lead to infants, reduced intake of protein, fat, vitamins, minerals.

Soft drinks aren't an appropriate alternative in the physician's opinion. The average teen male is consuming three to four cans of soft drinks a day. As teens consume more soft drinks, they get less milk and are at risk for osteoporosis (brittle bones) later.

Most American children and teens aren't putting on pounds because they are drinking too much milk even though dairy products are perceived as being fattening but doctors are stressing the need to families who are drinking whole milk to switch to non-fat milk.

For children who are overweight, eliminating caloric soft drinks and cutting back on fruit juice can have a beneficial effect. Children who cut back on juice can lose weight with little other changes because they are getting 800 to 1,500 fewer calories (a day). Eliminating sweet beverages has additional value in preventing spikes in the glycaemic index that make children hungry.

· To satisfy thirst both physicians and diet experts recommend giving children water. Water is thirst quenching and an ideal substitute if one wants to avoid making one's children overweight. Flavoured, non-caloric water is available and it is perfect!

The important rules to follow are:

1. Fruit juice should not be given to infants before six months of age. After six months of age, infants should not get juice from bottles or cups that allow them to consume juice easily throughout the day.

2. Infants should not get fruit juice at bedtime; putting a baby to bed with a bottle of juice can lead to tooth decay.

3. Children aged one to six should limit fruit juice intake to 4 to 6 oz (118-177 ml) a day.

4. For children ages seven to 18 juice intake should be between 8 and 12 oz (236-354 ml) a day. They should be encouraged to eat whole fruits.

These recommendations from the American Academy of Paediatrics (AAP) should be an ideal guideline for all the teenagers and parents who find it difficult to tackle the 'overweight' problem in their children.

Is Your Child a Fussy Eater?

Many children go through phases of being fussy eaters. This is a normal part of growing up. Children often want to eat a certain food in a certain spot at a certain time. They eat a small quantity of food and yet are well, active and growing normally. Most fussy eaters are between 1½ years and 5 years of age. Children of all ages commonly have a few food dislikes. Sometimes they dislike foods because of their colour but more

Serve nutritious food in attractive ways to make your child eat it.

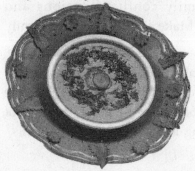
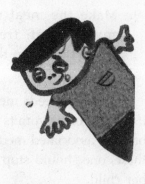

often because they are hard to chew. Children prefer well-cooked vegetables to raw vegetables. Modern research and experts recommend the following tips to manage a fussy eater:

1. Put nutritious food in front of your child. Don't worry on how much he is eating. It is the quality of the food that is important, not the quantity.

2. Drinking too much liquid can lessen your child's appetite. Limit liquid intake in the hour or two before meals.

3. Satisfy your child's sweet tooth by serving nutritious fruit-based desserts.

4. Avoid their snacking more than twice a day let them stick to a meal schedule. If your child doesn't eat at one meal, he will probably eat at the next.

5. Handle frustrating situations with patience, a positive attitude and firmness. Don't be aggressive or emotional.

6. Avoid power struggles—don't force feed plead, bribe your child.

7. Offer your child some choice in food and give small portions at a time.

8. Try serving food in attractive ways like cutting vegetables in odd shapes, decorating with ketchup or herbs.

9. Make the meal time table a relaxed and pleasant environment, free of family conflict, tensions and distractions like the TV. Make it an important family event.

The child needs medical evaluation if he is losing weight, if he gags on or vomits certain foods, if he is not active or if he has any associated medical problems. If the child has none of these, one should stop worrying and should not bother his/her child.

Weight Training Improves Figure

Many women are reluctant to train with weights because of the sometimes gruesome pictures of women who have acquired very masculine features due to anabolic steroid abuse. Unfortunately and often it seems this is an excuse to avoid a strenuous workout programme. For many women, however, this is an actual concern that prevents them from obtaining quality muscle tone, strength and fat loss. In reality, women do not have the hormonal make-up to support an excess of muscle mass or the hard masculine look associated with female body builders who abuse anabolic steroids. In fact, the average women will have to work much harder than the average man to acquire even a small amount of muscle. Fitness competitors seen in the magazines dedicate as much time in weight training at the gym as many top male body builders. Weight training benefits women by building a firm, curvy body rather than a bony, saggy body that crash diets and excessive cardio produce.

Also keep in mind that muscle burns calories throughout the whole day; so having more muscle will actually help keep the fat off. Forgetting what the crash diet programmes tell you is very important for looking good! Crash diets cause your body to eat your muscle because of inadequate nutrition.

A balanced diet composed of moderate portions of food from all food groups and a routine of weight training combined with cardiovascular exercise lead to the path to your goals.

If you do things the right way you can have a healthy life lead to style and look great without having to suffer or starve.

Modern research, medical experts, diet experts and beauty therapists all advocate the same principle— 'Eat and Burn'. Avoid crash diet programmes; instead eat properly and exercise which includes weight training also.

Midnight Binge

Americans have this bad habit of midnight binges. They get up all of a sudden in the night from their sleep, venture straight into the kitchen, open the fridge and start eating whatever is there in it—bread, cakes, fruits, cold drinks, soda, chicken, turkey, chips. After this midnight binge they are back to sleep. After sometime again they march to the kitchen and repeat the eating.

This midnight binge is repeated at least two or three times in a night. This habit has acquired the name 'midnight binge disease'. American research scientists warn the average weight Americans to stay away from this habit or quit it immediately if he/she has become addicted to it as it can lead to overweight and obesity.

It is alarming to know that what started in America is spreading slowly to other countries. Studies done in India reveal that this midnight binge has been found in India's cosmopolitan cities. With new brands of chips, colas and biscuits hitting the food markets everyday, it is not surprising to know that people are too tempted to try these new ones at least in a midnight binge!

NSRED

Nocturnal sleep related eating disorder

We have already seen a bit on 'midnight' binges.

Midnight munchies is a relatively small problem but NSRED is very serious. It is estimated that about millions of women have a condition called NSRED in which they consume large amounts of food during the night when they may be only half-awake. If they do remember they may be too ashamed to admit it in the morning. Pasta and sweet are favourites but on rare occasions people have been known to snack on cat food, cigarettes or cleaning products during their night time kitchen excursions. Other sleep problems such as sleep apnea, and restless-leg syndrome may prompt a binge episode.

The condition also has been linked to low melatonin levels and high levels of the stress hormone cortisol. Identifying the problem is critical, so treatment can begin and the person can take steps to avoid accidental poisoning, burning or cutting herself while preparing food for herself. If you are gaining weight and don't know the reason for it, you are inexplicably tired in the morning, and the kitchen which was clean when you went to bed, is now a mess if all these sound similar you are suffering from NSRED.

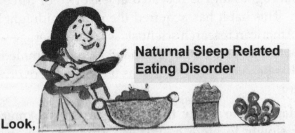

Naturnal Sleep Related Eating Disorder

Look,
how the appetite shines along with moon & stars

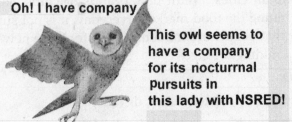

Oh! I have company

This owl seems to have a company for its nocturrnal pursuits in this lady with NSRED!

Is Nut Butter Better?

When we talk of butter, it is generally diary butter. Nut and seed butters, though commonly used in the West, are yet to conquer the taste of the Indian palate. When nuts and seeds are ground into a paste, they are referred to as butters. These butters are rich in protein, fibre and essential fatty acids. They are normally used as an alternative to diary butter or margarine and are eaten with bread or toast. Some of the nut butters can also be thinned and used in soups or as dips and sauces.

Commercial peanut butters may contain hydrogenated oil and additives but the natural ones are much healthier and are made purely from peanuts. Sesame seed butter (also called tahini) is also high in protein and used in Middle Eastern recipes.

Peanut butters are being made in Bangalore in India. They are made by a very simple process—peanuts are dried, roasted and crushed in a coffee grinder, that's all! A teaspoon of peanut oil is added when the process is started, but after the process starts the oil from the peanuts is itself the lubricant for crushing. No salt, sugar or additives of any kind are added. Yet the peanut butter has a shelf life of at least one-year!

Nutritionally one tablespoon of nut or seed butter has about 80 to 100 calories and 2.5 gm to 4 gm of protein. Nut and seed butters have 7 to 10 gm of fat in tablespoon mostly unsaturated fat. Nut and seed butters are good sources of many other nutrients including zinc, vitamin E, folic acid, copper, potassium. Most of these nutrients are not present in dairy butter.

Another important advantage over dairy butter is that nut and seed butters do not contain cholesterol. Nuts contain generous amounts of phyto chemicals that may be protective against heart diseases and cancer. Nut and seed butters are healthy choices when used in small quantities.

Ideas for Making Exercise Fit

When people vow to shape up with drastic actions like aerobics and dieting they must know certain important facts. To employ fitness to lose weight they must start with basic, 'big muscle' exercises before adding aerobics. And they must not diet until they have settled well with the exercise routine. Bob Greene, the man credited with helping Oprah Winfrey slim down, says if the above point is not followed, the person concerned may just slow his metabolism instead of boosting the caloric demands of his body. Greene advisses with stretching—to loosen the rusty muscles—then adding moves like sit-ups and stability ball exercises that strengthen shoulders, legs and abdominal. Those bigger muscles must be able to support the person concerned through running, biking and other aerobic activity. Also a sturdy foundation will help guard against back problems and joint strain. Greene's approach may not work everyone, says Walter R. Thompson, a kinesiology and nutrition professor at Georgia State University in Atlanta. He knows Greene and occasionally works with him. He feels that though Bob's concept may ease people into weight reduction, which is not a bad idea, people could easily fall off, the exercise regimen if they are not already convinced the combination of diet and exercise is the real key to weight reduction. The people's expectations of immediate results or early transformations are not possible. There are no shortcuts on the road to fitness and good health.

Good News in Chocolate

There is some good news about chocolate and nuts. But unfortunately the whole is not greater than the sum of its parts and there is still no good news about nutty chocolate, candy bars. Because chocolate is a plant it contains many beneficial plant chemicals including powerful antioxidants like flavinoids that may actually reduce the harmful effects of LDL, the bad cholesterol. These flavinoids may also reduce blood pressure.

Some animal studies credit cocoa flavinoids with reducing the growth of cancer cells.

While the amount of flavinoids in 2 oz of dark chocolate is about the same as that contained in a half cup of brewed black tea, those 2 oz contains almost 300 calories and 20 gms of fat. Having said that it is important to note that the fat in chocolate has little effect on blood cholesterol. Though it is highly saturated, the fat is mostly stearic acid, which does not boost cholesterol. Unfortunately, the logic only works if the fat you get from eating chocolates is a substitute for fat from some other source, not in addition to it.

Unsweetened cocoa powder, on the other hand, contains only 12 calories and 1.8 gms of fat. So while eating, chocolate can pack on the pounds, cooking with cocoa powder can give you the flavour plus valuable nutrients without the fat and calories.

Peanuts and other nuts such as almonds, walnuts, pecans, pistachios have now get a scientific licence. The scientific evidence suggests (that does not mean it proves) that eating 1.5 oz of most nuts such as peanuts as part of a diet low in saturated fat and cholesterol may reduce the risk of heart disease! The implication is that peanuts and other nuts contain specific components such as fibre, micronutrients and phyto chemicals that have been studied extensively and are thought to be important for chronic disease prevention. Peanuts are consumed maximum (among all the nuts) either as nuts, delicacies or as peanut butter. Other nuts in order of rate of consumption are almonds (next to peanuts these are consumed in high quantities), coconuts, pecans, walnuts, etc. Most nuts have 160-190 calories and 14 to 19 gms of fat per ounce; at least three-quarters of the calories come from fat. They are also among the best plant sources of protein. Nut butters have the same advantages and disadvantages that nuts do.

There are some nutritional differences between nuts:

1. Walnuts are rich in heart healthy alpha linolenic acid (an omega 3 fatty acid similar to those in fish);

2. Almonds are richest in calcium and vitamin E.

3. Brazil nuts are the best source of selenium of any food.

4. Macadamia nuts have the highest calories and fat.

5. Chestnuts have the least calories and fat (70 cal and 1gm of fat).

6. Peanuts are not true nuts but legumes (like dried beans). Similar nutritionally to nuts peanuts contain some Resvertrol, a beneficial compound found in grapes.

According to some studies, nuts also help reduce hunger longer than many other foods. An ounce or two a day will give the consumer the benefits and can easily be incorporated into a meal, instead of an extra snack. Chopped nuts are tasty in fruit or vegetable salads, yoghurt, oatmeal, home baked breads and muffins, pancakes, casseroles, breakfast cereal, chicken salad, rice dishes, stir fries. When possible nuts must be substituted in place of foods rich in saturated fat. Peanut butter is definitely a letter choice for a sandwich than cheese or most meats.

Low fat, relatively low caloric recipes can be made using nuts and chocolates. These can be beneficial to health serving both as a 'diet' and 'delicious' food.

Perils of Obesity

The overweight are particularly prone (and especially the mature female) to diabetes. The woman who has had several pregnancies with babies each of increasing size, or all of over average birth weight is well known to be at risk. It fact, the overweight and obese may by their size be demonstrating an essential inability to deal—an inability that later is shown in its more extreme form as diabetes. It has been said that overeating throws an excessive strain on the pancreas, a strain that in the end causes its failure. It may be however that those who become obese and consistently overeat are prone to diabetes through inheritance anyway. The evidence of control in diabetes by diet does show nevertheless; that a high blood sugar can be reduced and sugar in the urine eliminated by diet above, and this suggests that the cause and the effect are closely associated.

Obesity aggravates blood sugar level. In the recent times a lot of research has gone into this particular aspect. If a person is overweight and has type 2 diabetes, the doctor will urge him to drop those kilos knowing he will have a better chance of managing his blood sugar level. Today scientists are a bit close to knowing just why that's so.

A new study on mice suggests a fat- derived hormone called Resistin may promote insulin resistance, a condition in which the body fails to use insulin properly. Insulin controls blood sugar in the body. When there isn't enough of it or it isn't used effectively sugar builds up in the blood, starving the cells of the fuel they need for energy. Mice that don't have resistin are largely protected from insulin resistance suggesting new research. If resistin plays a similar role in humans, this finding could lead to new ways to and treat people with type 2 diabetes.

Burn Fat without Exercise

Japanese researchers claim to have found a way to get rid of excess fat without exercising, in a breakthrough that could lead to better treatment for obesity and diabetes. When a cellular receptor in muscles known as 'peroxisome–proliferator-activated receptor delta' or PPARd is chemically activated, it induces fat consumption in the muscle according to research led by Tokyo University professor of metabolic medicine, Juro Sakai. Receptors are proteins that translate a certain type of stimulus into nerve impulses. Calling PPARd 'a fat burning sensor', Sakai, who leads a research group at the elite university's research centre for advanced science and technology, said the finding offers "the possibility" of a drug that could end obesity. The drug could also be a treatment for diabetes as the PPARd activation also increased obese laboratory mice's sensitivity to insulin and helped reduce their blood sugar levels. The study found weight gain among mice given high fat feed whose PPARd receptors had been activated was about 40 per cent less than untreated mice on the same diet.

The activation of PPARd caused no excess weight loss as it worked less dramatically on non-obese mice, Sakai said. It did not trigger excessive eating either, he said.

37

Common Doubts Answered

Did you know?

In South India, especially Tamil Nadu, during the Navaratri festival, Godess Durga is worshipped as Shakambari, the one, who provides the entire universe with vegetables, fruits, grains and pulses. The idol of Durga is decorated with various vegetables, colourful fruits, different grains and pulses. Other food items are also used in the decoration.

When we see Durga decorated thus we cannot ignore the message conveyed so subtly: 'Have a well balanced diet with vegetables, fruits and grains in right amounts.'

---

1. *Just about everyone we meet are on a diet or about to go one. Isn't this 'overdoing' the reducing business?*

No! People reduce for all the wrong reasons—mostly for looks/cosmetic reasons. They fail to realise that obesity is a major health hazard. Obesity leads to disease and death. What is wrong about reducing is not how much we do but how we do. Practically every reducing diet, no matter how well it works at the start, is doomed to fail after a few weeks.

2. *Do many diets have a common basic fault?*

Yes! Any diet that changes the pattern of our natural eating habits is physiologically unsound and therefore unacceptable to our body. Most fads diet work—for a short time. But after a few weeks, one is forced to give them up, and any weight lost is promptly regained. Scientific studies show that approximately 45 per cent of our daily food calories come from fats, 40 per cent are derived from carbohydrates and 15 per cent from proteins. One can tolerate minor variations in these ratios but not drastic changes. One doesn't need a university education to select a balance diet; one can let one's natural desires lead them. Selection of the right ratio is built in mechanism. Sedatives, stimulants and appetite depressants are ineffective suggest conservative doctors. The weight loss they reduce is merely transitory and once they are stopped, the weight is regained.

   3.   *Are low calorie foods an aid to reducing?*

'Not really! Filling our stomach with low calorie foods won't satisfy our hunger. Only sufficient calories can do that. Most people mistakenly believe that when the stomach is full, hunger is satisfied. The control on hunger is in a group of cells located at the base of our brain (hypothalamus area) called <u>Appestat</u> which functions more like a thermostat or automatic regulator. When the amount of sugar in our blood drops below a fixed level, the appestat clicks on and signals hunger. Then when the levels rises to a certain point, the appestat registers satiety and click off.

   4.   *If the amount of food or calories we eat is automatically regulated by the appestat, why are some people fatter than others?*

That is still the big unknown. Obviously, a fat man's appestat must switch on and off at a higher setting than a thin man's. Why, we don't know. Nor do we know how to change the sitting, explain the endocrine specialists.

   5.   *Then attempts to reduce seem doomed to fail, why try?*

It is hopeless only if one tries to reduce by fooling his appestat or radically altering his natural eating patterns. One can control one's weight successfully by applying a basic principle learnt in school physics—the conservation of matter. By merely changing the word matter to energy and we have the answer to weight control. (The original law is matter cannot be created or destroyed. It can be only transformed from one form to another. Here, substitute the word matter with the word energy.) This concept can be called Energetic. Our bodies transform the food we eat into energy which we use to maintain life processes and to perform our daily activities. The energy we do not use immediately is stored as body fat for future use.

Food, as everyone is aware, contains varying amounts of calories. Recently scientists have been able to count the number of calories our bodies use in performing basic function as well as in various sports and work activities. Since all foods and activities now have caloric equivalents, we can keep daily count of the calories we eat and the calories we expend.

6. *How does one know how many calories can be taken?*
The formula sounds simple:

    a) To maintain body wt = keep calories eaten and those spent in perfect balance.

    b) To gain body wt = eat more calories than those spent.

    c) To reduce body wt = eat fewer calories than those burnt up.

The answer lies in by using this equation:

3,500 calories equal about half a kilo of body fat, thus if a person sets a goal to lose half a kilo a week, his calorie intake for that period must be at least 3,500 cal less than his caloric expenditure. When he eats fewer calories than he expends his body takes the needed calories from stored body fat, thereby reducing his weight.

7. *When we cut down our calorie intake, can we eliminate the most fattening foods?*

If we do, we will commit the same error that makes all fad diets fail: altering our basic eating pattern. Although some foods are more fattening than others—for example, fats contain more than twice as many calories per units as carbohydrates or proteins—we should not stop eating fats; just reduce our overall calorie intake.

8. *Then energetic is not strictly speaking a diet but rather a method of controlling weight?*

True. We do not change our way of eating. When mealtime comes, we eat the foods we like; merely regulating the amount.

9. *It seems that there are two ways to control weight with the above concepts of energetic (1) the amount of calories we consume (2) the amount of exercise we do.*

Yes. Ideally we should combine the two. For instance, to lose about half a kilo a week, we can reduce our calorie intake by 1,400 and increase our expenditure by 2,100. On a daily basis we can accomplish the goal by doing without three slices of bread and by taking a brisk 60-minute walk.

10. *Is exercise self-defeating? Activity also increases the appetite; so does that mean exercise is a poor way to lose weight.*

Not so. Exercise does stimulate appetite and will increase eating but not enough to account for the calories burned. Tests on individuals prove that vigorous exercise for half an hour a day will produce a weight loss despite increased food consumption. The usual ratio between exercise and increased eating is about 800 calories expended and 500 taken in, leaving, deficit of 300. There are some hard working men who eat as much as 6,000 calories a day more than twice the usual amount, without gaining weight!

11. *Suppose a woman wants to take two kilos off her hips and thighs. How can she do this by above-mentioned 'energetic' method?*

She cannot do it with any method. Spot reducing is an illusion. Exercising one set of muscles or having them jiggled with some machine will not reduce the fat from that area. However, it will improve muscle tone and perhaps appearance. When stored fat is burned, it is taken from all over the body, not just where the activity exists.

12. *What exercises are better than others in burning stored fat?*

There are two answers to this question: what is ideal and what is practical. Ideally, the more vigorous the exercise, the more fat it will consume. But how many people can play tennis for an hour? Or go swimming regularly? Practically one must pick the activity that is most convenient, a brisk walk, exercises in one's room, using stairs instead of lift, in short, anything that will make the person breathe hard.

13. *Suppose a man wants to lose 15 kilos. How long should it take him with energetic?*

Most patients who lose weight readily have an easier time maintaining that loss. Reducing gradually is the best way according to many medical experts. If 15 kilos is our goal, we must take off the initial 2½ kilos during the first month. This weight must be maintained for an additional month and the next month another 2½ kgs must be reduced, and so on. Using this system a person can lose 15 kilos a year and keep them off.

14. *With energetics, controlling the weight seems to be like balancing one's bank account. Deposits are the foods we eat. Withdrawals are our activities and how they balance out is the statement of our weight up, down or even. Is this interpretation correct?*

Exactly. We must start by writing down our expenditures,

expressed in calories according to the values given in charts (refer the section on useful charts). We must include everything we do each day while at work, at home or at play. We must also make note of every morsel of food we eat or drink for a week and then average the total to a daily basis. The difference between intake and output will indicate how much we must decrease our food calories and increase our activities to achieve the weight we want.

15.   How can an unhappy dieter make his life a bit more bearable?

Unfortunately, a dieter must live his life a little on the hungry side. However, the burden can be eased. Many reducers make the mistake of saving almost their entire allowance of calories for the evening meal when their activities are at an all time low and consequently, many of these calories will be stored as body fat and not burned. Instead, dieters should spread their intake of food calories more equally throughout the day to match the calories used in their daily activities. By doing this, all the calories they eat will be burned by their job and reaction and will not be stored. As a matter of fact, if a person is going to reduce, he must forget the three meals a day routine. He would do better as a nibbler than as a gobbler.

16.   What is this so talked about 'S-Factor'?

S-Factor refers to the 'strength training', reshaping the body by working out with calisthenics, small weights or resistance equipment. Strength training is a dieter's dream, because for every kilo of flab that a person replaces with muscle he burns dozens of extra calories per week. The reason is that muscle tissue is more metabolically active, muscle cells have more chemical reactions than fat cells do. A 70 kg person whose weight is mostly leans can eat 500 calories more per day than someone of the same weight who is largely flab. And this doesn't count the calories burned by the workouts

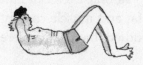

- PUSH UPS
- OVERHEAD PRESS
- TRICEPS EXTENSION

- LATERAL RAISE
- LOWER BACK
STRENGTHENER

Includes
. LUNGE
. CALF RISE
. CRUNCHES

Note:
These Exercises must be done
only with the guidence of a Fitness Expert
There are 2 or more steps Involved.
Needs slow and steady movements.

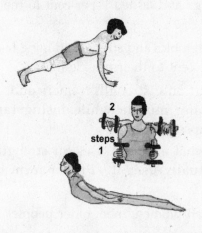

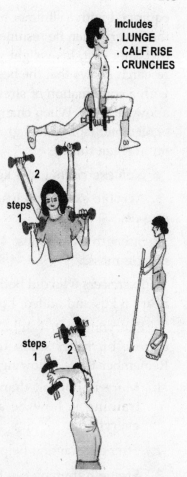

themselves—a typical section will expend more than a hundred. Once the person is in shape, the S-factor may let him eat 25 per cent more than before.

By contrast people who don't exercise lose about a quarter kilo of muscle each year. The calories that would have been burned by muscle end up being stored as fat. That's what causes middle age spread. Crash diets are even worse. These accelarate muscle loss, because the body attempts to ward off starvation by burning lean tissue as well as fat. The person equipped with a slimmer but flabbier body gains more weight than ever, when he resumes normal eating. Result: as he tries diet after diet, his weight yo-yos higher and higher. Medical research shows that the best way to beat middle age spread is with a combination of strength training, aerobic exercises and a low fat diet. When changes in body fat and muscle content of 65 dieter (split into 4 groups) were studied, the results were on average thus:

Non exercisers lost 4 kgs but 11 per cent of it was muscle.

Aerobic exercisers lost 4½ kgs but only 1 per cent was muscle.

Strength trainers lost 4 kgs and added 9 per cent to their muscle mass.

Exercisers who did both aerobics and strength training lost neary 6 kgs and added 4 per cent to their muscle mass.

Everyone lost weight but only strength trainers added calorie-burning, body-toning muscle while losing fat. Remember these following tips:

1. More important than what a person uses for strength training is how he actually uses it. Proper form is everything.

2. Strength training helps all women, men, older people.

3. Strength training can be done at home or in health clubs.

4. Strength training isn't time consuming. Workouts can take as little as 20 minutes.

5. Workout should include a minimum of eight exercises that use the major muscle groups.

6. One can try strength training two or three times a week 20 to 60 minutes of aerobic exercise three to five times a weak. One can do both in the same session and on alternate days.

7. Each movement has to be performed slowly and steadily for maximum benefit.

8. A fitness expert or a medical expert's opinions can be taken before starting for proper guidance.

17. Obesity is one of the leading causes of accelerated aging. Is it true?

Yes! If a person loses weight, stops smoking and exercises he can slow the aging process and make dramatic changes in his looks in a relatively short period of time. Good nutrition, plenty of rest, exercise everyday, inclusion of raw fruits and vegetables in diet, a positive attitude (quit worrying) all these lead to improved quality of life, good looks and a check on the aging process. Let us discuss some aspects here:

1) **Skin:** When a person's weight fluctuates, the skin stretches with the weight gain cycle, but it may not completely shrink back to its original size in the weight loss cycle. As a result the skin may sag.

A well balanced diet with ample supplies of nutrients is thought by many experts to produce a glowing, younger look. Zinc, vitamin A, vitamin C are all important for skin. The diet should include greens, seafood, fruits and juices, tomatoes, red and green peppers, broccoli, 6 to 8 glasses of water for adequate hydrating.

2) **Hair:** Healthy, shining hair is second only to vibrant skin for making one look younger. Unbalanced diet affects hair. Some people in their obsession to lose weight quickly go on a fad diet, high in fibre and bulk, but low in protein. Over a few months, they lose a lot of weight but along with this a good deal of hair is also lost! When diets don't contain enough amino acids (the building blocks of protein) there is a dramatic increase in hair loss as the body breaks down its own protein. Hair and skin cells are constantly reproducing and are very sensitive to nutritional deficiencies. Grains,

legumes, meat, eggs and milk are foods rich in amino acids and must be taken in appropriate quantities.

Nutrition experts recommend the following important rules for a healthy, look younger diet:

a) Vitamins C, E, beta carotenes known as antioxidants are important for slowing down/preventing ailments associated with aging and to boost the immure system.

b) Key to good general nutrition is balance. Proteins should make up roughly 10 per cent of daily calorie intake. No more than 30 per cent should come from fats. They remaining calories must come from complex carbohydrates preferably.

c) The average diet however contains too many fats and sweets and not enough fruits and vegetables. This should be rectified.

d) The fat in fried foods, whole milk diary products, cakes, worries and red meat is one of the biggest culprits. There must be a definite cut back on one's fats and salt and sugar must be used in moderation. The effects of aging can be showed by paying closer attention to nutrition . There is mounting evidence to support this statement. 'Age fast or Age slow—it is upto you' declare health experts. Age,

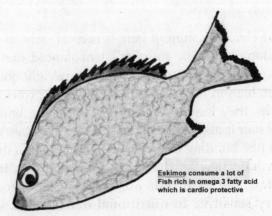

Eskimos consume a lot of Fish rich in omega 3 fatty acid which is cardio protective

related declines in physiological function seem to have less to do with aging than with environmental factors like diet and exercise. With proper planning and execution of diet and exercise one can stay healthier and youthful.

18. *What are the various positive points in the diet and food habits of various cultures and countries, which can be included in designing a perfect balanced diet?*

i) **The Mediterranean Connection**—People who live in the countries bordering the Mediterranean have in general impressive health and longevity. Some features of their cuisine—the reliance of fresh fruit, vegetables and wholegrains, for instance—fit current concepts of a healthy diet. But other features don't. For example, scientists have been puzzled by a health mystery popularly known as the 'French paradox'. The French consume at least as much saturated fat as the Americans, yet the death rate from heart disease for French men are only about 40 per cent of that of the American men. Some researchers attribute this protection from heart disease largely to the consumption of Wine. In south-western France the average man drinks two to three glasses of wine (mostly red) every day with meals.

When many people think of Mediterranean cuisine, they immediately picture garlic and onions. Modern science is finding surprising medicinal powers in these related bulbs, which contain many organic sulphur compounds. Garlic has blood thinning properties like that of aspirin.

Several epidemiological studies in China have pointed to reduced stomach cancer risk in those eating diets rich in vegetables of the onion family.

ii) **Asian Wisdom:** Green tea enjoyed in Japan is a popular 'pick me-up' food items. It has many antioxidants offering protection against cancers. Japanese men smoke twice as much as American men yet they have only about half the lung cancer mortality. Perhaps the fact that Japanese drink green tea daily helps explain why. Soya beans have been a staple diet in East Asia for thousands of years. Soya bean paste soup and its protective power against gastric cancer has been established by some researches. Soya bean cured called tofu, soya milk, soya flour, soya protein isolates, Soya sauce all contain anti cancer agent and are to be included in our diet.

iii) The Arctic Diet: Eskimo diets include abundant fish salmon, mackerel, herring, and others—rich in unusual oils that scientists label omega 3 fatty acids. It consumed for a long time. These fish oils thin the blood, decrease cholesterol, reduce inflammatory reactions decrease risks of cancers and atherosclerosis. More coldwater fishes have to be included in diet.

19. We want to know about 'anorexia nervosa'.

Anorexia nervosa was given its name by Sir William Gull in 1874. Although he described its clinical feature among them, emaciation, amenorrhea, constipation, and oedema of the legs—he made No mentioned of 'weight phobia' as a motive for self-starvation. He suggested that the loss of appetite was the result of Mental perversity. It was not until the 1930's that the German term for the illness 'Mager Sucht' or 'addiction to thinness was coined. According to psycho historian R.C.C.Asper, the drive towards thinness does not emerge as a common and predominant motive until 1960." The modern psychiatrists diagnostic and statistical manual lays down the criteria for anorexia nervosa which can be summed up as:

   a) Intense fear of becoming obese.

   b) Refusal to maintain normal body weight.

   c) Weight loss of at least 25 per cent.

   d) Disturbance of body image, i.e., a distorted attitude towards one's own body shape and weight (dysmorphophobia).

e) Anorexia often goes hand in hand with bulimia which is characterised by binges, i.e., eating large amount of food within a short span of time. In India the 'morbid fear of fatness' is considered a crucial criterion of anorexia. This is rare in anorexia of non-Western countries and cultures. There is a link between Westernisation and fear of obesity. Anorexia in non-Western cultures reflect family pathology. Anorexia is a family stress response pattern specially related to parental conflict child's distress due to family problems, and stress may take the form of anorexia. Here it seems to act as a regulator!

20. *What about the genetic basis of obesity?*

Researchers say that the discovery of gene that causes obesity in mice when it is defective is a major breakthrough that opens a new basis for understanding energy regulation in people and also about obesity. The researchers reported that they have for the first time isolated a gene in mice that is involved in the normal process of regulating weight and that a similar gene found in the humans may play the same role. This finding is a major breakthrough because it gives researchers a powerful tool that regulate body weight, said Nobel Prize winning neurobiologist, Torsten Wiesel, president of the Rockefeller University in New York, where the discovery was made several years. This can also lead to the possibility of devising new drugs to treat obesity, a serious disease that can predispose people to such life-threatening condition such as diabetes, heart disease, high BP. But researchers warn that such human treatments are years away and would only be possible after a series of scientific discoveries. Research indicates that 60 to 90 per cent of the variability in people's weight can be attributed to genes with factors such as diet and exercise accounting for the rest. The newly discovered mouse gene called 'ob' for obesity regulates fat storage in the body. It does this by making fat cells secrete a protein that signals the brain to suppress appetite or alter energy metabolism when the body has enough fat. When muted in mice the 'ob' gene no longer delivers its appetite, suppressing protein signal, and the mice develop a syndrome that resembles extreme obesity and type II diabetes in humans. The team has also found that an 'ob' gene in humans causes the production of a protein identical to mouse protein but not the same.

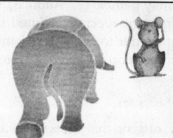

For problem as big as 'his' body (obesity) these scientists have discovered the gene in 'me' of all the beings! Funny! Isnt it?

NEWS: The 'ob' gene discovered in mouse regulates fat storage in the body. Ob stands for obesity!

21. *What are the important points to remember in weight gain in pregnancy?*

The average woman gains 12.5 kg during pregnancy. Though a normal woman may lose weight or gain over 20 kg, Much of the increase is accounted for by the

    a) Uterine contents.

    b) Enlargement of maternal organs.

    c) And also particularly in the third, trimester-increased body water.

The remainder average about 3.5 kg is fat. By a not fully understood mechanism pregnancy alters the carbohydrate metabolism and subcutaneous fat is laid over the abdomen, back, and upper thighs mainly in the first and second trimester. The fat is usually lost again afterwards, a process aided by the loctation and for most women long-term weight gain is an effect of age rather than parity. Never the less during pregnancy fat women tend to put on more weight than thin ones. Women who are overweight at the start of pregnancy face an increased risk of complication. Hypertensive disorders are more frequent, though the incidence in different report varies widely—from 7 per cent to 46 per cent. Abnormal glucose tolerance is more common, affects 7 to 17 per cent of women. Increased risk of urinary tract infections and possibility of thromophlebities have also been reported. But the risk of anemia and protein delivery may be lower than in underweight women. Recent studies don't confirm the point that parental mortality was high among obese women. Obese women tend to have large babies. Dietary restriction cannot be advocated even in the obese primigravida (first time pregnant) as it is possibly detrimental to the baby and of no benefit to mother. But a decrease in weight of obese women is important.

22. *There is so much 'hype and hoopla' on fibre diet. What is it and what are its advantages?*

A generation ago it was called as roughage and was recommended as a cure for constipation. Today, it is called fibre and aids in preventing constipation. It also has other benefits. Foods rich in fibres can lower blood pressure and cholesterol levels and they thus decrease the risk of heart attacks. They can also help to lose weight. Dietary fibres can prevent or treat intestinal diseases and cancers. They also help in treatment of diabetes. Fibres are easy to get, as many foods contain abundance of fibres? Non-vegetarian foods appear fibrous and are tough to chew. But this is misleading. What are dietary fibres? The answer is dietary fibres are that part of the plant that one's body cannot digest. What our body needs is vegetable or plant fibre. It is of various varieties and is found more in unrefined and raw foods. Overcooking destroys fibres. There are two main types of fibres:

1. Those that are soluble, and

2. Those that are non-soluble.

Both play different but important roles in promoting health. Soluble fibres include pectins, gums, and mucilages. These form gel-like substances in the intestin and are useful in preventing and treating heart diseases and in controlling diabetes and hypoglycaemia. Good sources of soluble fibre include oats, barley, chana, lentils, carrots, green peas, couliflower, pears; non-soluble fibres include hemi-cellulose, cellulose, lignins, add bulk to the stool and speed elimination. They help to prevent and /or treat intestinal disorders such as constipation and irritable bowel syndrome and possibly cancers of the colon, prostate, breast, ovaries. Good sources of non-soluble fibres are wheat, corn, bran, whole wheat breads, beans, nuts, seeds, popcorn, fruits and vegetables. The last mentioned are particularly very rich in fibre, if eaten raw with peel.

23. *How does obesity become a risk factor for children?*

Low fat diets have proved to be safer and healthier food for growing children. Overweight is a serious disease of appetite regulation and energy metabolisms affected by a combination of genetic, cultural, social, economic, psychological and environmental factors. Obesity which is defined as an "important, chronic, degenerative disease that debilitates individuals and kills prematurely" is on the rise among children. Being overweight is directly related to diabetes, high BP, heart disease, cancers, gall bladder disease, gout and osteoarthritis. Fatty lesions can develop into atherosclerosis in children as young as three years old! Children eat more but there has been a decrease in active lifestyle. Lack of physical activity is the main factor in causing obesity. One- fourth of our children already have the cholesterol levels of 170 or more. Children spend more time in passive TV watching, computer, videogames. After smoking obesity- related conditions are the second most common cause of death in the USA. Risk factors in the childhood produce heart disease in adults. Producing a healthy breed of children with obesity free body requires two measures (1) low fat diet (2) encouraging an active lifestyle.

24. *'An apple a day keeps the doctor away' says an old dictum. What does the modern research say about this?*

Consumption of fruits and vegetables reduces the incidence of cardiovascular disease and cancer according to a study by researchers from the London School of Hygiene & Tropical Medicine. The researchers estimate that 2.6 million people die per year due to inadequate fruit and vegetable intake. Consuming 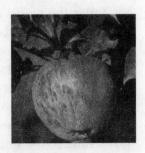 around 600 gms of fruits and vegetables every day can reduce the incidence of heart disease by 31 per cent, heart strokes and stomach cancer by 19 per cent and lung cancer by 20 per cent 'An apple a day keeps the doctor away' has been authorised even by modern researchers!

25. *What is the new concept of "nutraceuticals" all about?*

Medicine was always food in traditional diets. But now science and industry are rediscovering this ancient knowledge. This modern science of nutraceuticals is here to revive the diet lifestyle linkage and to curb the 'pop new pills everyday' culture. The idea that food has therapeutic value is not a new one. Ayurveda, for instance, recommends diet regimes based on seasons and on individual constitution. Traditional communities in most countries had dietary practices that placed a premium on nutrition. But then the world changed. We moved from eating home cooked and seasonally grown vegetables to diets that are much more fashionable and convenient: vegetables come out of season; food moves across regions; traditional grains disappear. At the same time diseases such as obesity, diabetes, cancer, asthma—now seen as lifestyle diet related—increased and science began to rediscover the traditional wisdom of food as medicine.

But food in its natural form made poor business, so industry isolated compounds like immunity boosting polysaccharides from *Curcuma longa* (tamarind) and found a new delivery system—pills, tonic, powders, syrups.

Enter the world of nutraceuticals. Nutraceutical is defined as food or parts of food that provides health benefits including prevention of disease. The nutraceutical industry makes these health foods in attractive form and packages them in eye-catching, user-friendly ways. Are nutraceuticals food or drugs? Certain health claims for food are allowed as long as the claim was based on authoritative statements by a governmental scientific body. Antidiabetic powders, dietary supplements, traditional drugs all are making their own claims under the 'nutraceutical' label to get sanction as food or food product. But products sold as tablets, capsules are not food, say nutraceutical-regulating bodies. At present a lot of confusion prevails in this 'nutraceutical' classification. Traditional systems of medicine like ayurveda, unani, siddha have different rules and regulations and their products, drug recipes, processes and ingredients need a separate classification and sanction. What one needs to learn at present is (1) The use of food for therapy is an integral part of traditional medicine. Modern medicine also has many 'food as medicine' recommendations to make. (2) 'Nutraceuticals' based on the principle of using food to provide health benefits concerns with the industry making food products in various forms and delivery system. But nutraceutical 'products' are yet to be properly classified, authorised and approved. (3) Many of the nutraceutical products, lifestyle and diet, could help in obesity treatment.

26. What is NES?

NES is Night Eating Syndrome. Midnight binges and nocturnal sleep-related eating disorder all are variations of this NES. US researchers found that normal weight people with the condition of Night Eating Syndrome, resembled obese people with NES in their eating habits and other behaviours except that people with NES who were obese were almost nine years older than non-obese night eaters. Furthermore,many obese night eaters reported that they believed their tendency to snack at night preceded their weight gain. People with NES typically wake up between one and four times each night and snack on about 300 calories worth of food. They are sleep deprived as a result, or feel frustrated that they cannot control their cravings. They are typically conscious of their eating habits. In contrast, people with other types of night eating problem will snack while sleep-walking and are often unaware of their behaviour. Approximately 1.5 per cent of the population has NES but the condition has been found in up to 15 percent of the people who are obese. In non-obese night eaters this syndrome leads to weight gain and obesity after a while.

27. How can a pot belly be corrected?

The pot belly is made up of 3 layers:

1. outer fat 2. middle muscle 3. inner distended intestines.

Reducing the pot belly thus involves losing fat, toning up the lax and sagging muscles of the abdomen and developing correct eating habits to improve intestinal tone and reduce distension. People usually associate pot bellies with extra fat and focus all their attention on losing weight. However, the quickest way to reduces a pot belly would be to take up the lax abdominal muscles (at the same time working up a weight loss programme and correcting eating habits). On self-pinching the waist generously for every ½ inch pinched above one inch, he is probably overweight by 10 pounds; he must lose weight at the rate of ½ kg/week, not more than that. There are some ways to lose weight:

1. Starting the meal with two to three raw vegetables and glass of watery soup without flour or cream and thin buttermilk also is included in this meal. Only one cereal

at a time with either pulses or cooked vegetables, for e.g.,
roti and vegetable or rice and dal. The moment a person
feels full, he must stop eating.

2. Replacing one major meal, lunch or dinner with
   vegetables (a cucumber, a tomato, a carrot, for
   instance) and three fruits. These will not only fill up
   but also give nutrients, vitamins and minerals of a
   balanced diet.

3. A flour must be prepared that contains equal
   proportions of wheat, rice and green gram. This flour
   is rich in vitamins, protein, fibre, calcium, iron,
   electrolytes. It is easiest digestible even when eaten
   raw. This flour can be mixed with water, curd, milk
   or coconut water to be made into a paste. Some spices,
   finely cut vegetables can be added or even fruits can
   be added. One big bowl is ample substitute for either
   lunch or dinner.

We have already discussed the exercises for reducing pot
belly. Abdominal exercises includes crunches, twisted
crunches, hip and leg raise, twisted leg and hip raise. The
abdomen is worked in six parts—upper centre upper right,
upper left, lower centre, lower right, lower left. These exercises
will yield results.

The digestive system must be subjected to at least some
unrefined food every day. If this unrefined food forms 25 per
cent of our daily diet in the form of raw vegetables, fruits,
distention would be reduced, intestinal tone will improve and
consequently the pot belly would be remedied. Regular hours
of eating, proper chewing of food are also important for a
proper eating habit.

Nutritionists say?

1. Olive oil and canola are best for cooking. Flaxseed oil is
   the best source of essential fatty acids but is to be avoided

in cooking as heat changes flsaed oil into a toxic derivative known as lipid peroxide.

2. Only fish that is broiled or baked actually protects against heart disease. Fish sticks don't count. Fried fish contains only small quantities of Omega 3 FA—the healthy fat that can improve cholesterol and other cardiac factor. Only 'Baked fish' for heart advise scientists.

28. Which is the healthy oil for cooking?

We must avoid oils like coconut oil and palm oil for cooking as their fat content is too much. Sunflower oil contains PUFA (Pollyunsaturated fatty acids). But if eaten in large quantities they can cause gallstones. Sunflower oil has important advantages. It decreases cholesterol but increases HDL and protects against heart disease. Olive oil, sesame oil, etc., contain MUFA (monounsaturated fatty acid). Sunflower oil etc., has PUFA. So a mixture of 65 per cent of olive oil/sensame oil with 35 per cent sunflower oil is ideal for cooking. Whatever be the oil used the amount consumed should not exceed 30-50 ml/day.

It is true that refined oils are harmless. These are oils which have been refined by removing unwanted dirts, etc., and their colour, taste are suitably altered to suit our tastes. They are advertised as 'cholesterol free' which is not true. So one should never believe the claim that refined oils are perfect for health.

29. Are Bakery products good for one's health?

Bakery products are the favourites of many people. To increase the 'crispness' and to make it 'crunchy' vanaspati is added in generous amount to many bakery products. When the vegetable oils are hydrogenated, harmful fats are formed. These are more dangerous than the fat of meats. The heart is affected by such fats. Moreover, in bakery products, wheat is avoided and maida is used. Adding insult to injury is the high fat content of creams used in cakes. These also contain high sugars. The cheese used in pizza also can increase cholesterol and pave the way for heart attacks.

Thus these high in sugar, high in fat bakery products are to be consumed in small quantities once in a while. They are meant only for a small bite or munch.

30. Can the Mediterranean diet improve arthritis?

A recent study showed that arthritis sufferers who followed the Mediterranean diet had up to 38 per cent less pain and stiffness and hand weakness. Fruits, vegetables, olive oil, fish and chicken seem to have a beneficial effect on arthritis inflammation.

31. Many people complain of gaining weight despite exercise. How does this occur?

The most common reason for weight gain is simply that more calories are being consumed than calories being burned. Exercise will not help a person lose weight if he does not change his eating habits. People assume that just because they are exercising they will automatically lose weight. But even if we do several hours of vigorous exercise every day, and eat more than we burn, we will still gain weight. People believe that whatever excess calories they eat today they will be able to burn tomorrow by doing more exercise than normal. Many people cheat themselves by not giving their all when they exercise. They spend a lot of time in a gym but most of the minutes are spent chitchatting! Others are working out at very low intensities when they are capable of burning more calories. So the frequency and duration of their workouts is appropriate but the intensity is sorely lacking. Other people think they are exercising regularly when in reality their workout attendance is few and far in between.

It is possible to become smaller in measurements but gain weight on the scale because one is losing fat and gaining muscle. This happens especially when people do weight training. But some people are so weight conscious that even if they lose inches, they are not happy because they weigh a few pounds more than others. They need an attitude adjustment: otherwise, they may quit exercising, thinking it is not worth it when they are really on the right track.

Charts, Tables and Sample Diet

Protein, Fat, Carbohydrate Content of Different Foods

Food	Protein %	Fat %	Carbo-hyrate %	Fuel value per 100 gms/ calories
Apples	0.3	0.4	14.9	64
Asparagus	2.2	0.2	3.9	26
Bacon, Fat	6.2	76.0	0.7	712
Broiled	25.0	55.0	1.0	599
Beet, medium	17.5	22.0	1.0	268
Beets, fresh	1.6	0.1	9.6	46
Bread white	9.0	3.6	49.8	268
Butter	0.6	81.0	0.4	733
Cabbage	1.4	0.2	5.3	29
Carrots	1.2	0.3	9.3	45
Cashewnuts	19.6	47.2	26.4	609
Cheese, cheddar, American.	23.9	32.3	1.7	393

Food	Protein %	Fat %	Carbo-hydrate %	Fuel value per 100 gms/ calories
Chicken, total edible	21.6	2.7	1.0	111
Chocolate	(5.5)	52.9	(18.0)	570
Corn (maize), entire	10.0	4.3	73.4	372
Haddock	17.2	0.3	0.5	72
Lamb, leg, intermediate	18.0	17.5	1.0	230
Milk, fresh, whole	3.5	3.9	4.9	69
Molasses, medium	0.0	0.0	(60.0)	240
Oat meal, dry, uncooked	14.2	7.4	68.2	396
Oranges	0.9	0.2	11.2	50
Peanuts	26.9	44.2	23.6	600
Peas, fresh	6.7	0.4	17.7	101
Pork, ham, medium	15.2	31.0	1.0	340
Potatoes	2.0	0.1	19.1	85
Spinach	2.3	0.3	3.2	25
Strawberries	0.8	0.6	8.1	41
Tomato	1.0	0.6	8.1	4.1
Tuna, canned	24.2	10.8	0.5	194
Walnuts, English	15.0	64.4	15.6	702

Note: High proportions of fat and proteins in meat product and high proportions of carbohydrate in vegetables and grains.

The following list tells how many calories a person burns per hour at various activities. With this information, plus a calorie chart, one can balance calorie intake against expenditure.

Job Activities

Answering telephone	→ 50
Bathing	→ 100
Bed making	→ 300
Brushing teeth or hair	→ 100
Dressing, undressing	→ 50
Driving car	→ 50
Dusting furniture	→ 50
Eating	→ 50
Filing (office)	→ 200
Gardening	→ 250
Ironing	→ 100
Mopping floors	→ 200
Light gymnastics	→ 500
Painting	→ 150
Piano playing	→ 75
Rowing	→ 400

Recreation

Badminton	→ 400
Basketball	→ 550
Card playing	→ 25
Cycling slowly	→ 300

Soccer	→ 650
Swimming leisurely	→ 400
Running fast	→ 900
Skating leisurely	→ 400
Skating rapidly	→ 600
Skiing	→ 450
Walking upstairs or downstairs	→ 800
Washing up	→ 75
Swimming rapidly	→ 800
Tenpin bowling	→ 250
Tennis singles	→ 450
Tennis doubles	→ 350
Preparing food	→ 100
Reading	→ 25
Sawing	→ 500
Sewing	→ 50
Typing	→ 50
Cycling (strenuously)	→ 600
Dancing slow step	→ 350
Dancing fast step	→ 600
Fishing	→ 150

Golf   → 250
Hiking   → 400
Horse riding   → 250
Singing   → 50
Running slowly → 600
Walking leisurely → 200
Walking fast   → 300

Ideal Weight Chart for Men and Women
Age group: 22 to 25 years
Frame: small to medium built
Unit: kilograms

Height	Weight (men)	Weight (women)
5'2"	50.5 to 58.5 kg	46.5 to 54
5'3"	52 to 61 kg	47.5 to 55
5'4"	53.5 to 62 kg	49 to 57
5'5"	55 to 63 kg	50.5 to 58.5
5'6"	56 to 65 kg	52 to 61
5'7"	58 to 66.5 kg	53.5 to 63
5'8"	60 to 69	55 to 65
5'9"	62 to 71	57 to 66.5
5'10"	63.5 to 72.5	58.5 to 68.5
5'11"	65 to 75	61 to 70
6'0"	67 to 77	63 to 72
6'1"	69 to 79	-
6'2"	71 to 81.5	-
6'3"	72.5 to 84	-
6'4"	74 to 86	-

For women in the height range of (small to medium build)

4 feet 10 inches   Ideal weight can be 42 to 48.5 kg

4 feet 11 inches   Ideal weight can be 42.5 to 50 kg

5 feet   Ideal weight can be 43.5 to 51 kg

5 feet 1 inch   Ideal weight can be 45 to 52.5 kg

2. **Required**   **Daily Amounts of the Vitamins**

Vitamin A   5000 Iu.

Thiamin (B_1)   1.5 mg

Riboflavin (B_1)   1.8 mg

Niacin   20 mg

Ascorbic Acid (Vit C)   45 mg

Vitamin D   400 Iu

Vitamin E   15 Iu

Vitamin K   none

Folic acid   0.4 mg

B_{12} 3 Mg

Pyridoxine (Vit B_6)   2 mg

Pantothenic acid   unknown

Iu   → *International units*

Mg → *Micrograms*

mg → *Milliegrams*

a) Markets are full of diet plan books offering model diet for weight reduction.

b) Before adopting any such diet one should seek a doctor's view and a trained dietitian's expert opinion also.

Diet Plan

Offers 1,200 calories per day

This is a model diet plan, a very strict one.

Note: The 5-meal pattern. This diet plan needs a diet expert's approval before adoption.

- **Early morning**: one glass of warm water with few drops of lemon juice added to it.

- **Morning Breakfast**:

  One small fruit

  (Or)

  One single slice of bread

  (Or)

  Two or three small tomatoes or cucumbers.

  Note: Any one of the above item can be taken (or) two of the above items can be taken.

- **Mid-day Lunch**: First one cup of green leaf soup can be taken; then

  1. One small bowl of vegetables

  2. Two small chappatis.

  3. One small bowl of moong or any similar cereal can be consumed.

  Note: Flour should not be used for preparing soup.

  · Non-vegetarians can take some lean meat or a fish.

- **Afternoon or Early Evening**

  One cup of milk without sugar or one cup of tea or coffee with a little milk (sugar to be substituted with artificial sweetener).

  One small fruit

  (or)

  Two or three small tomatoes or cucumbers

  (or)

One slice of bread

Note: One or two of the above items can be taken. Those who take eggs can take one egg as one of the item. They can take one egg and one small fruit.

- **Night or supper:** First clear vegetable soup can be taken. (no flour added),

    One small bowl of rice or khichdi.

    One small bowl of vegetable.

    One small bowl of moong or similar cereal can be taken.

Note: Non-vegetarians can take some lean meat (without fat) or a fish.

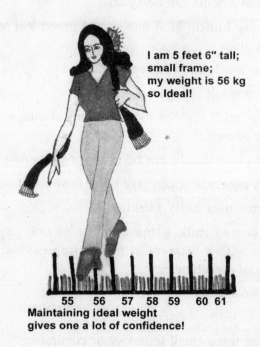

I am 5 feet 6" tall; small frame; my weight is 56 kg so Ideal!

55 56 57 58 59 60 61
Maintaining ideal weight gives one a lot of confidence!

Bibliography

1. Textbook of _Medical Physiology;_ Guyton.
2. _Diabetes_ (pocket health guide)
3. _Know your body_ (2nd Edition)
4. Oxford Hand Book of Clinical Medicine.
5. Medical Journals
6. Newspaper reports
7. Research information from medical reports, magazines.
8. Certain medical sites were broused on internet to get the latest update on certain aspects of obesity.